SO-AKF-570

Living Well with Dystonia

OUTDATED MATERIAL
WITHDRAWN

RC 935 .D8 T78 2010
Truong, Daniel,
Living well with dystonia

SANTA MONICA COLLEGE
LIBRARY
1900 PICO BLVD.
SANTA MONICA, CA 90405-1628

Living Well with Dystonia

A Patient Guide

DANIEL TRUONG, MD
MAYANK PATHAK, MD
KAREN FREI, MD

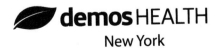

demos HEALTH
New York

SANTA MONICA COLLEGE LIBRARY

Acquisitions Editor: Noreen Henson
Cover Design: Gary Regalia
Compositor: NewGen North America
Printer: Hamilton Printing

Visit our website at www.demosmedpub.com

© 2010 Demos Medical Publishing, LLC. All rights reserved. This book is protected by copyright. No part of it may be reproduced, stored in a retrieval system, or transmitted in any form or by any means, electronic, mechanical, photocopying, recording, or otherwise, without the prior written permission of the publisher.

Medical information provided by Demos Health, in the absence of a visit with a healthcare professional, must be considered as an educational service only. This book is not designed to replace a physician's independent judgment about the appropriateness or risks of a procedure or therapy for a given patient. Our purpose is to provide you with information that will help you make your own healthcare decisions.

The information and opinions provided here are believed to be accurate and sound, based on the best judgment available to the authors, editors, and publisher, but readers who fail to consult appropriate health authorities assume the risk of any injuries. The publisher is not responsible for errors or omissions. The editors and publisher welcome any reader to report to the publisher any discrepancies or inaccuracies noticed.

Library of Congress Cataloging-in-Publication Data
Truong, Daniel
    Living well with dystonia: a patient guide / Daniel Truong,
Mayank Pathak, Karen Frei.
        p. cm.
    Includes index.
    ISBN 978-1-932603-23-1
    1. Dystonia--Popular works. I. Pathak, Mayank. II. Frei, Karen. III.
Title.
    RC935.D8T78 2010
    616.8'3—dc22

                                                      2009051551

Special discounts on bulk quantities of Demos Health books are available to corporations, professional associations, pharmaceutical companies, health care organizations, and other qualifying groups. For details, please contact:

Special Sales Department
Demos Medical Publishing
11 W. 42nd Street
New York, NY 10036
Phone: 800–532–8663 or 212–683–0072
Fax: 212–941–7842
E-mail: rsantana@demosmedpub.com

Made in the United States of America
10 11 12 13   5 4 3 2 1

To my friend, Victor Passy, whose loyal friendship I cherish; To Richard Obosky, Victor and Janie Tsao, Hedy Orden, Suzanne Mellor, Robert Farmer, James Ruetz, Khalique Khan, Greg Jones, and Donald and Darlene Yoshikawa, for whose support I am grateful; to all my patients from whom I've learned so much.

—DDT

To Bharti, who accorded me time, patience, and tolerance.

—MSP

To all my dystonia patients who have taught me as much as I have treated them and to Justin and Vi of the NSTA for their unending and tireless dedication helping those with dystonia.

—KF

Contents

Foreword

Dystonia is a life-altering disorder. No question about that. And it has changed the lives of hundreds of thousands of Americans. The earliest symptoms of dystonia begin subtly and may initially be dismissed as the result of fatigue or a minor injury. Understandably, concerns rise as the symptoms persist or get worse. Many people receive the diagnosis after numerous visits to different physicians. They go from doctor to doctor, explaining over and over again what is going on with their bodies. Finally, a diagnosis emerges, and this moment is usually the first time people have ever heard of this disorder: "Dys-to-nia-what?" Now they know what it is called, but what is it?

Living with dystonia often means learning to live in a new body. It may mean learning to manage a great deal of pain—pain that often limits what you can do. It may mean having to give up simple daily activities or changing your career.

And yet, many people who have been diagnosed with dystonia have not allowed it to control their lives. They have discovered new areas of interest and found new activities that they can enjoy with family and friends. They have resolved to learn more about their bodies and to educate themselves on what dystonia is and how it is treated. After the initial shock and concern over the diagnosis, they come to discover that they are stronger and more resilient than they thought. These persons are an inspiration to all of us.

Studies have shown that when people managing a chronic condition educate themselves, they do better. When you take the time to learn all you can—especially from the conversations you have with your doctor—you become an active part of your own treatment plan.

Treating dystonia is an art as well as a science. What works to relieve symptoms for one person with dystonia may not work for another. It may take a couple of tries to discover the most beneficial treatment plan. You and your doctor must work together to find what works best for you.

We hope you will use this book as a resource for you and your family. It is a tool to help you become better educated about your dystonia and the breadth of available treatments. It provides an overview of what dystonia is, how it is diagnosed and treated, and suggestions on what other things you and your doctor might consider doing to help you with your dystonia. Get informed, stay informed, and get connected. Join a support group or find a forum online. And know you are not alone in this. These steps will help you in your battle with dystonia.

Janet L. Hieshetter
Executive Director
Dystonia Medical Research Foundation

Preface

Twenty years ago, dystonia was not a well known disorder, even to neurologists. But, thanks to the efforts of patient organizations, it is no longer obscure and has even developed into a subspecialty of neurology. It is, however, still vaguely recognized by most physicians who are not neurologists. Many of our patients lived with their disorder for years before receiving a definitive diagnosis. Additionally, there remains a lack of information outside of the professional medical literature for use by affected individuals and their families. It is for this reason, to develop educational and reference materials appropriate for laypersons, that we wrote our first book, *The Handbook of Spasmodic Torticollis*, in conjunction with the National Spasmodic Torticollis Association. That book, intended for persons afflicted with one particular type of dystonia (spasmodic torticollis, also known as cervical dystonia), sold well. In recent years, the understanding of dystonia and its treatments have markedly expanded. *Living Well With Dystonia* includes expanded sections on the various forms of the disorder.

This book provides comprehensive information for patients with all kinds of dystonias and the people close to them. Medical terms and concepts are introduced sequentially and then used as building blocks for the later discussion. Although we have provided an extensive glossary, we suggest that you read the chapters in order.

Our intent is to present a clear definition of each dystonia, categorize it appropriately as a movement disorder that is part of the broader category of neurologic diseases, and differentiate it from other conditions with which it may be confused. We discuss different types of dystonia and present the relevant anatomy and physiology of the nervous system. We have drawn on the stories of our patients to build a progressive depiction of the experiences an individual might have as he or she goes through the initial onset of symptoms, progression of the disorder, finding good medical care, receiving a diagnosis, undergoing treatment, and subsequent outcome. Personal vignettes from the experiences of selected patients are provided to illustrate particular points in the discussion. Subsequent chapters discuss various modes of treatment for dystonia. Chapters 13 and 15 are largely reprinted from our previous book.

Prior to the mid-1980s, there were no specific treatments for dystonia. Nearly all treatment consisted of using oral medications that were primarily intended for other medical conditions. Most of these medications are still in use, and a few new ones have been added. Chapter 10 details and discusses the general principles of medication therapy. During the past decade, a more specific intervention, chemodenervation using botulinum toxin, has become the primary and most effective treatment for some forms of dystonia. More familiar to the public as a cosmetic treatment for wrinkles, there is little awareness of botulinum toxin as a treatment for movement disorders. We have addressed this problem in Chapter 11. Additionally, for those few patients requiring deep brain stimulation surgery, we provide a description of neurosurgical techniques in Chapter 12.

Chapter 15 is a manual of therapeutic rehabilitation exercises. Our patients repeatedly ask us if there are any exercises or rehabilitative techniques they can follow to help alleviate their symptoms. For these reasons, we developed a group of exercises that can be performed by most patients without assistance and using a bare minimum of equipment. We first presented these exercises in a videotape, *Physical Therapy and Exercises for Spasmodic Torticollis.* In this book, we present these exercises in the same order and format used in the videotape. This book may be used alone to learn the exercises or in conjunction with the videotape.

Since each person's case of spasmodic torticollis is different, only certain exercises are appropriate for them. We advise you to read through each of the exercises in the chapter. Each exercise contains a description of the particular muscles and type of abnormal neck position that it is intended to treat. You can thus identify which exercises are appropriate for you and discuss the exercises with your physical therapist if you have one. Please obtain permission from your doctor before beginning any of the exercises. The figures in this book were drawn by Dr. Mayank Pathak and Dr. Hiep Truong, who have strived to accurately represent subtle differences that pertain to different forms of dystonia without making the drawings either too complex or too simple.

Daniel Truong
Mayank Pathak
Karen Frei

A Tribute to Mattie Lou Koster

In 1986, I had a chance to share a bus ride to a dystonia retreat outside of New York City with a remarkable woman. I was a fellow in my first year in Movement Disorders, a new field of neurology. The motherly woman who spoke with a Texan drawl gently told me the story of a life with blepharospasm. I do not remember now how long the bus ride was. For me it went quickly as she was such a fascinating, inspiring woman. I learned so much about blepharospasm from her. She was an amazing woman with a disarming gentle charm.

After being diagnosed with blepharospasm in 1980, Mattie Lou Koster of Beaumont, Texas, decided to found the Benign Essential Blepharospasm Research Foundation (BEBRF) at the age of 68. In addition from suffering from the symptoms and associated difficulties of the disorder, she had recently lost her husband of 50 years. Koster was subsequently diagnosed with leukemia, breast cancer, and peripheral neuropathy. She later underwent a mastectomy and two hip replacements. Indeed, Koster was an amazingly courageous and resolute woman who overcame many obstacles to fulfill her mission of advancing knowledge about blepharospasm and providing support to people with the disorder. Koster was extremely dedicated to the BEBRF. She knew she was not the only person dealing with blepharospasm and wanted to help others with the disorder. With the knowledge that blepharospasm patients at the time felt isolated and struggled on a daily basis to deal with their symptoms, Koster founded the BEBRF with the intent to help them and to make the disorder more widely known. She was so dedicated to helping people with blepharospasm that, even as the BEBRF expanded, she had calls directed to her personal phone when the office lines were not open so that she could immediately assist anyone who needed help. The organization was originally run from Koster's home office, where she wrote and mailed newsletters and took calls. For the first six years, the BEBRF was staffed entirely by volunteers and supported only by small donations from locals and Koster's own funds.

The BEBRF eventually became widely renowned due in large part to Koster's efforts. She wrote to a number of medical schools throughout the United States to request more information on blepharospasm and also spoke to any doctors who crossed her path. The first major advance Koster made in spreading knowledge about blepharospasm was when she gave a 10-minute speech to the American Academy of Ophthalmology. The next day, she attended the first of many press conferences that would make an increasingly greater number of doctors aware of blepharospasm. For the same reason Koster also appeared at physicians' meetings nationwide and subsequently introduced many doctors to using botulinum toxin to treat blepharospasm. She even volunteered to be the first human subject to undergo an experimental procedure developed by Dr. Jonathan Wirtschafter, called chemomyectomy. It involved a series of injections around the eye to paralyze some muscles permanently and theoretically reduce or eliminate blepharospasm symptoms.

Another of Koster's achievements was to bring together blepharospasm patients from around the world. The newsletters, pamphlets, and other materials that her organization published were influential in making contact with many people with the disorder.

When shipments of botulinum toxin were suddenly suspended and blepharospasm patients were left without any form of treatment, Koster wrote an article in the BEBRF newsletter to encourage her readers to write to the U.S. Food and Drug Administration to resume distribution of the toxin. She managed to organize many people affected by blepharospasm around an important cause and eventually shipments of botulinum toxin resumed.

Another significant occurrence that united blepharospasm patients was when the *Wall Street Journal* published a front-page article on the disorder in January 1982. Suddenly hundreds of people realized that blepharospasm was the cause of their symptoms and many physicians learned of the disorder for the first time. Koster was also very successful in organizing symposiums about blepharospasm. She always made sure to invite doctors that specialized in either ophthalmology or neurology, since both subjects are relevant to blepharospasm. This provision also ensured the opportunity for neurologists to interact with ophthalmologists and vice versa, which in turn generated ideas about better treatments for blepharospasm.

Mattie Lou Koster was a forceful and motivated woman who devoted all of her time and energy to the BEBRF and its mission of helping blepharospasm patients and distributing information about the disorder. Her efforts allowed the BEBRF to rise from its humble origins to become an invaluable resource to all people with blepharospasm.

Daniel Truong

Acknowledgments

The authors have not personally suffered with any type of dystonia; we thus acknowledge and give profuse thanks to our patients, whose personal accounts of their illnesses have lent this book a personal touch from a first-hand perspective.

We also acknowledge and thank those of our patients who gave us their personal experiences to use as vignettes, and all of those and their loved ones from whom we have gleaned knowledge over the years. Our special thanks go to Donna Ball, Barbara Barry, Wanda Glaze, Brita Goldsmith, Kathrin Hogan, Dave Jones, Greg Jones, Khalique Khan, Edward Kho, Suzanne Mellor, Ruby Netzley, Lee Ann Orrick, Leslie Rodriguez, Jim Ruetz and Jenine Flood-Ruetz, Dot Sowerby, Darlene and Kristi Yoshikawa for their stories.

We also thank Dr. Hiep Truong for drawing the pictures in Chapter 7.

1

Introduction

If you are reading this, you or someone close to you has probably been diagnosed with some type of dystonia. Dystonia can take many forms, but all are characterized by involuntary muscle contractions that lead to abnormal postures or involuntary repetitive movements. Dystonias are relatively uncommon disorders, and many physicians— even some neurologists—don't know much about them. Patients with some dystonias are often misdiagnosed at least once. Patience and perseverance are important in getting an accurate diagnosis and the best care.

Gathering information is the first step in managing any chronic disorder. Finding a specialist in movement disorders or in treating your kind of dystonia, educating yourself about your disorder, and talking to other people with the same diagnosis are all essential to finding the best treatment and achieving the best quality of life.

In this book we provide both the patient's perspective and the medical perspective to help you begin educating yourself about dystonia. You will learn about factors that may cause dystonia, the signs and symptoms of the condition, how it progresses, and how it is treated. This book will serve as a reference for you to share with your doctor and family.

In our years of treating patients with disabling neurologic conditions, we have found that over several years patients seem to triumph over their initial feelings of despair and adapt to their new state of health and ability. You will see examples of this in the "Patient Perspective" sections of some chapters.

Newly diagnosed patients have the most difficulty coping with dystonia. It used to be that they got a 'cold' and, when the condition went away, they would get back to being themselves. Now they are faced with something permanent. It is not easy to accept this new reality. The following story is shared by a patient who now takes her condition in stride.

PATIENT PERSPECTIVE

At 60 years of age, I now have a very different perspective on my illness than I did when I was 36, when my symptoms first started. Back then, I didn't know what dystonia was. If asked, I would have guessed dystonia to be an obscure, small, Eastern European country. Yeah . . . that was then. I was so young, so innocent, so . . . not used to the pain I would have to learn to live with.

A lot has changed since 1984: year-one "BC" (before cervical dystonia). I have adapted. That is what I do. I adapt. I don't fight it; that makes it worse. I don't curse the fates anymore; they are obviously deaf. I don't ignore it; that definitely does not work. I just adapt, take it on the chin, go with the flow, hop on the bus.

I will share my list of why's with you. A "why" is really just a "why the heck me and not someone else?" You may pick the one you think is the correct answer, if you like.

1. *My parent hit me in the head one time too many.*
2. *I had convulsions as a child.*
3. *My sibling landed me in the hospital with a broken clavicle, broken rib, ruptured spleen, and slight concussion.*
4. *I'm Irish and an Ashkenazi Jew.*
5. *I was in the car in the middle of the five-car crash, and I was the one who got whiplash.*
6. *It's my uncle's fault: he had Parkinson and that's in the same family as cervical dystonia.*
7. *I was in a very unhappy marriage for a very long time and was very depressed when the symptoms started. This would make it my first husband's fault; a plausible "why" for many.*
8. *Rare disorders gravitate to me. I can be pretty interesting on paper, if you are a doctor.*
9. *I had a near-death experience.*
10. *It is written.*

Actually, my symptoms may have started as early as my childhood. I had a twitch in my right eyelid. Everyone said it was because I was nervous. That twitch has come and gone throughout my entire life. Maybe there is something to that?

"BC" I lived a pretty healthy, normal life. I mean that I was not a street urchin or a hermit. I had not done drugs, didn't go to Woodstock, and was probably considered boring. There came a time though, when, just like in a movie, when all the planets align and everything comes crashing down, I found that very thing happening in my very own life. I had always been the strong, dependable, capable one and I was changing into an anxious, depressed, squirming, self-conscious agoraphobic. It was as if I had been possessed. I no longer had control over my body, my feelings, and I felt very lost, ugly, and alone.

I saw doctors. I saw doctor after doctor. It's disturbing to be at the mercy of someone who is just as helpless as you are when it comes to doing anything at all to change what you are going through. I was told that I had chronic upper back muscle spasms, that I needed to take more iron, that I was suffering from anxiety as a result of being an adult child of an alcoholic. On and on it went. Nothing changed except that the disease got worse. I was at an all-time low. I couldn't drive. I was embarrassed to go out and be seen with my tremor and my head pulled almost to my shoulder. I was crying every day, and felt more and more pain as time allowed the muscles in my neck and back to twist, pull, and torture me.

It was 15 years ago when I saw a doctor who said he knew of a doctor who might know what my condition possibly could be. I was jaded: I'd been burnt before. But I was hopeful.

Now, Dr. X is quite the character. Once you get to know him you understand his genius. He became my BFF (best friend forever) as soon as he circled my frightened self while I sat quietly in that office chair listening to him list off the symptoms I had been living with for several years. It was unnerving to hear someone so absolutely right. After that, it was just taking care of business.

Learning I had cervical dystonia was overwhelming at first, yet the feeling of vindication was marvelous. Living with it has been a lifelong challenge. I've morphed back and forth through surgery and injections of botulinum toxin. I've educated myself. I've shared some of my time and talents in hopes of making a small difference to others with the disorder. I have even met and married a man who has dystonia. That part was not a sacrifice. He's the best thing that has ever happened to me.

Yes, at the age of 60 I do know a lot more than I did at age 36. I have learned how fragile we are, how helplessness can change into empowerment when you work with dedicated and compassionate people. I have no regrets regarding my inability to enjoy some of the "normal" things many others my age take totally for granted. I'm very grateful that for some reason known only to doctors, they decide to find out "why" and "what can be done" to help people in need. My life would be so different and so much more limited if I had not been fortunate, if I hadn't crossed paths with my BFF and so many other kind and caring souls. Maybe "It is written."

Not everyone with dystonia has this patient's attitude. She moves on and her dystonia becomes a side show, not the main event. Because we admire her attitude, we decided to share her story with you. We hope that the information in this book will help you to achieve your goals and to get the answers you need to live the best life possible with your dystonia.

In the following chapter, we will walk you through a basic under-standing of the nervous system, an overview of the different types of dystonia, methods of diagnosis, and treatment. The two subsequent chapters discuss the genetics of dystonia and related diseases or other factors that can cause it. The five chapters after that discuss different dystonia syndromes in detail. Descriptions of different forms of dystonia are intertwined with real life stories. There is a chapter on oral medicines used in dystonia treatment. Botulinum toxin injection, a mainstay in the treatment of dystonia symptoms, is given its own chapter, followed by a chapter on deep brain stimulation, which is becoming the standard of treatment in certain dystonia syndromes. Cervical dystonia, a complicated and relatively common form of dystonia, is allotted a large chapter of its own. A final chapter on coping with the diagnosis and symptoms of dystonia is followed by a section on therapeutic home exercises and appendices listing support groups and other information.

2

Overview of Dystonias

THE NERVOUS SYSTEM

Dystonias are neurologic disorders. Specifically, they are movement disorders, meaning that they are caused by dysfunction of the motor part of the nervous system, and result in some abnormal involuntary movement. The nervous system includes the brain and spinal cord, known as the *central nervous system*, as well as all the other nerves in the body, known as the *peripheral nervous system*. There are two types of nerves in the peripheral nervous system: those that bring sensory information from the body to the brain (sensory nerves) and those that bring motor information from the brain to the muscles of the body (motor nerves) (Figure 1). Sensory nerves carry information about touch, pain, taste, vision, and other sensations. Motor nerves carry signals to muscles that cause them to contract.

To understand how sensory and motor nerves work, consider this scenario: if you touch a hot stove, sensory (pain) information is sent via sensory nerves in your finger up through your spinal cord and into your brain. The brain then sends signals down the spinal cord and out through the motor nerves to muscles that pull the hand away from the stove.

The brain contains billions of nerve cells called *neurons*. Neurons send and receive information among one another using electrical and chemical signals. The motor system is composed of certain brain areas, their neurons, and their information pathways which receive and send information. In dystonia, signals from motor neurons are abnormal, causing uncontrollable muscle contractions that lead to abnormal head, limb, or body postures and/or movements.

Here is a simple example of how the muscles produce joint movements and postures. Your elbow joint works very much like a simple hinge. It can bend or straighten when it is pulled in a certain direction. The major muscle that bends the elbow is the biceps,

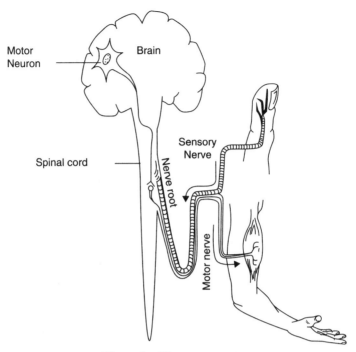

Figure 1   *The nervous system.*

a group of muscles in the part of the arm above the elbow. When your arm is straight and relaxed, the biceps muscles are loose and elongated (Figure 2). When you want to flex your arm, the motor system in your brain sends electrical signals through your spinal cord and into motor nerves that enter the biceps muscles. When the electrical signal reaches the biceps, the biceps muscles become "excited," which causes them to contract, or to shorten. When they shorten, they pull on the arm bones that they are attached to. Since the shoulder is attached to the trunk and can't bend toward the elbow, the muscle contraction causes the elbow to bend, drawing your forearm and hand toward your shoulder (Figure 3).

Now, back to the big picture: when you are awake, all the muscles in your body are experiencing a low level of electrical excitation; this is known as resting tone. Resting tone is caused by constant, low-level signals from the motor system in your brain. Resting tone allows you to maintain your body posture and balance, and keeps your muscles ready for voluntary movement when you need it. This occurs unconsciously: your brain constantly adjusts the resting tone of your muscles to your situation, whether you are sitting, standing,

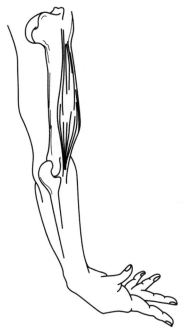

Figure 2   *Biceps muscle relaxed at full length.*

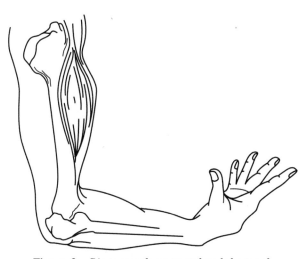

Figure 3   *Biceps muscle contracted and shortened.*

or lying down, and how alert you are. The brain "knows" when to make these adjustments based on information (feedback) from the sensory nerves in your muscles and joints, the balance mechanisms in your ears, and visual information received through your eyes. As when you touched the hot stove, sensory input relays information to the brain that it uses to modify position, movement, and posture.

The motor system is divided into two subsystems: the primary (*pyramidal*) motor system and the secondary (*extrapyramidal*) motor system. The primary motor system (Figure 4) consists of neurons in the gray matter on the surface of the brain that send out signals for movement along wire-like extensions known as *axons.*

These axons run deep into the brain, through the brainstem, and down to the spinal cord. From there, the signals (information) are relayed to another group of motor neurons (secondary motor neurons), which then send the signals out through their own axons along the motor nerves, and finally to the muscles.

At first glance, it would seem that the primary motor system should be all that is needed to move your arm or any other body

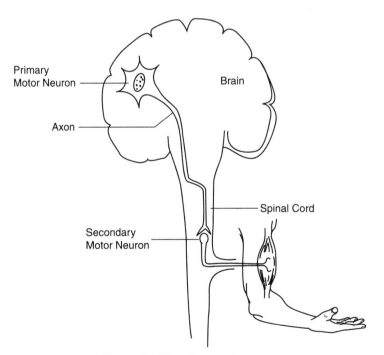

Figure 4   *The primary motor system.*

part, but control of movement is not so simple. Not only are you able to will your arm to lift or your hand to grip, but also to control the distance you move your arm, the speed at which you move it, and the amount of force you exert with your arm or your grip. For example, the amount of force needed to grip and lift a doughnut is less than what is needed to lift a dumbbell.

The regulation of all movements and the constant little adjustments that must be made during movements are the responsibility of the secondary (extrapyramidal) motor system. The main components of the extrapyramidal system are called the *basal ganglia* (Figure 5). These are a group of nut- and berry-sized clusters of neurons located near the center of each half of the brain (together, certain of the basal ganglia are sometimes referred to as the *striatum*).

The basal ganglia receive and integrate information from sensory nerves and organs, such as the eyes and ears. The basal ganglia have extensive connections allowing communication with the pyramidal motor system and almost all other areas of the brain. The basal ganglia use the sensory input to fine-tune the output of the pyramidal motor system to allow you to accomplish tasks as different as hammering a nail and threading a needle. The basal ganglia are

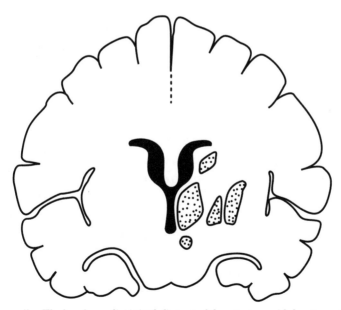

Figure 5   *The basal ganglia (stippled), part of the extrapyramidal motor system, deep in the brain.*

critically important to controlling the resting tone of muscles. They also prevent excess or unwanted movements by reducing uncontrolled pyramidal output.

Dystonias are often called *extrapyramidal disorders* or *basal ganglia disorders*. The neurons of the basal ganglia communicate among each other and with other parts of the brain through their axons. The ends of these axons release chemicals that act as messengers to the next cells in line and determine the response of that neuron. These brain chemicals are known as *neurotransmitters*. The basal ganglia neurons use a number of different neurotransmitters, including *acetylcholine* and *dopamine*. Medical conditions or drugs that interfere with the normal action of acetylcholine or dopamine may result in movement disorders. A deficiency of dopamine can result in muscular rigidity, increased resting tone, and/or a reduction of normal movement; excessive dopamine can lead to an increase in undesired movement such as tremor, twisting, writhing, or abnormal posture.

Dystonia, as previously explained, is one type of movement disorder. Different movement disorders affect the motor system in different ways. For example, in Parkinson disease, movements are slowed down, and limbs or other body parts become stiff and exhibit a shaking tremor. In dystonias, muscles involuntarily spasm and contract, pulling or contorting the affected body parts into abnormal postures. Sometimes, the affected body parts also exhibit tremor, writhing, or even flinging movements. These movements are called *dyskinesias*.

The muscle contractions of dystonia can affect one muscle or many, manifesting symptoms in different parts of the body, including the head and neck, face, eyelids, voice box, hands, or even the whole body. However, involuntary and sustained muscle contractions that cause abnormal postures, twisting of a body part, and/ or repetitive movements are common to all dystonias. There may or may not be pain associated with the movements and muscle spasms. Dystonia does not affect intelligence, and it is not a psychiatric (mental) disorder. Dystonias are generally progressive. Early on, dystonia symptoms are intermittent and more likely to happen during the performance of some activity or movement, or during stress. Over time, symptoms may become more severe or frequent, and may occur even when patients are walking or relaxing.

CLASSIFICATION OF THE DYSTONIAS

Dystonias are often classified according to the pattern of involvement of body parts:

- Generalized dystonia affects most or all of the body.
- Focal dystonias affect a localized part of the body (e.g., the neck, the arm, etc.).
- Multifocal dystonia affects two or more unrelated body parts.
- Segmental dystonia affects two or more parts of the body next to each other.
- Hemidystonia affects the upper and lower limbs on the same side of the body.

Table 1 lists the different types of dystonia and their classification by pattern of body-part involvement.

Another way to classify dystonias is by whether they are *primary* or *secondary*. Primary, or *idiopathic*, dystonia appears "out of the blue", with no obvious cause; about half of all dystonias are of this type. Some idiopathic dystonias are inherited or otherwise genetically programmed, but the precise cause of most cases of idiopathic dystonia is not known. Primary dystonias may also be further classified by the particular genetic defect, if known, that produces them. However, most patients with primary dystonia do not have an identifiable genetic defect. The known genetic defects produce a minority of dystonias. The genetics of dystonia are discussed in Chapter 3.

Secondary, or acquired, dystonia is caused by disease or some environmental agent that damages the basal ganglia. Secondary dystonia can be caused by a number of things, including infection, drug reactions, poisoning, trauma (brain damage from injury), stroke, or complications at birth. These causes will be further discussed later in the book. Most of the dystonia types listed in Table 1 can be primary or secondary in nature.

DIAGNOSIS OF DYSTONIA

As the patient stories in this book make clear, the symptoms of dystonia may be subtle early in the course of the disease. Stiffness, movements, tremors, and pain may be attributed to overuse or strain of a body part, tendon or joint problems, or simply stress. Because

Table 1   *Classification of Dystonia*

Name of Dystonia	Location of Dystonia	Area of Dystonia
Blepharospasm	Eyes	Focal
Oromandibular dystonia	Mouth, may also include tongue	Focal
Meige syndrome	Eyes, mouth, meck	Segmental
Spasmodic dysphonia	Voice box	Focal
Cervical dystonia	Neck	Focal
Writer's cramp	Hand	Focal
Trunkal dystonia	Trunk	Focal
Oppenheim's dystonia		Generalized

dystonia is relatively rare, primary care physicians may not at first recognize mild cases as neurological conditions. If the neck, head, or face is involved, the patient may be suspected of having a psychiatric disorder.

Doctors may recommend rest, ice, heat, massage, or physical therapy. They may prescribe pain relievers, balms or salves, and muscle relaxant medications. In mild cases, these conservative measures may be all that are needed to make the symptoms tolerable or acceptable, even if the definitive diagnosis of dystonia is not made. If the disorder progresses over time, however, these interventions will become ineffective, and more blatant movements and postures will declare the presence of a serious underlying condition. At this point, the patient should be referred to a neurologist.

During the interview, a neurologist will try to ascertain the presence of factors in your medical history known to cause movement disorders. These might include a history of birth complications that can result in brain injury. Other historical factors include brain infection during infancy or later, previous head injury affecting the brain, or a known history of stroke. Any event during which the brain is deprived of oxygen (*anoxia*) at any point in a person's life may produce dystonias. Such episodes may include near drowning, smoke or fume inhalation, choking or other causes of asphyxiation, cardiac failure such as occurs during a heart attack, or the prolonged respiratory failure that can occur in drug overdoses. In order to produce a permanent movement disorder, the anoxia must be severe enough and prolonged enough to produce coma for some length of time.

It is especially important for the diagnosing physician to know whether the patient has ever been admitted to a psychiatric facility, has been under any psychiatric care, has received chronic treatment for gastrointestinal disorders of nausea or dysmotility, or has otherwise been exposed to neuroleptic (antipsychotic) medicines. In our practice, past exposure to neuroleptic drugs is the single most common cause of a neurologic condition that looks almost identical to primary cervical dystonia. Some examples of medications that can cause such disorders are Haldol, Risperidal, Zyprexa, and Reglan. If other potential causes of dystonia are not found during the interview, the physician should suspect the presence of a primary idiopathic movement disorder.

There is generally no blood or other laboratory test or imaging study that will diagnose primary dystonias. The abnormality affecting the basal ganglia in dystonia is chemical or functional in nature. It is, therefore, not visible on conventional brain imaging studies such as *computed tomography* (CT) or *magnetic resonance imaging* (MRI). The diagnosis is made when a neurologically experienced physician obtains a detailed history from the patient regarding the onset and progression of the symptoms, and then performs a careful physical exam. MRI or CT imaging may be ordered to exclude other brain conditions that may mimic or induce dystonia. The physician may also order blood tests to look for other medical conditions, some of which are discussed in Chapter 4, that can cause secondary dystonias. Finally, in selected patients, genetic testing may be done to see if one of the known causative genetic defects is present. For these reasons, a person suffering from dystonia may not receive a firm diagnosis the first time they are seen by a doctor. Often, a person with dystonia will be seen and treated by many different doctors for years before receiving the definitive diagnosis.

It is usually a neurologist who makes the definitive diagnosis: most neurologists have enough experience with dystonia to recognize it and initiate treatment. Even in a general neurology practice, however, dystonia cases make up only a tiny fraction of the patient population. Whether a neurologist is able to provide more advanced treatments for dystonia depends on the concentration of patients in his or her practice. Therefore, a neurologist will sometimes refer patients who do not respond well to treatment, or those who have severe or complicated cases, to a subspecialist in the field of movement disorders.

Neurology clinics specializing in movement disorders are mostly found at major university medical centers, although some neurologists specializing in movement disorders practice at private medical centers, in private groups, or independently in the community.

TREATMENT OF DYSTONIA

A number of treatment options are available for managing the symptoms of dystonias, but there is no one treatment that works in every type of dystonia or for every patient, and there is currently no cure. Treatments include oral (by mouth) medications, injections with botulinum toxin, surgery, and rehabilitation therapy. Treatment is individualized, and it may take your doctor several tries to find the best medication or other treatment option for you. Sometimes a combination of treatments, such as oral medication and botulinum toxin injections, may produce the best control of symptoms. You will need to work with your doctor to develop the appropriate treatment regimen for your dystonia.

Some medicines do not treat the dystonia itself but are used to treat associated symptoms, such as pain and depression. Pain medicines can be taken orally, injected into muscles that are in spasm for temporary pain relief, or be delivered into the fluid that surrounds the spinal cord by means of an implanted pump. Other oral medications suppress the dystonia by affecting either the central nervous system or the muscles themselves. Oral medications are not curative; they only suppress the symptoms. Generally, such medicines cause only a moderate reduction of the dystonic muscle spasms. Further, they have troublesome side effects, such as drowsiness or dry mouth, which limits the dosage that can be used. These medications affect the entire body, not just the parts suffering from dystonia. Oral medications will be discussed in detail in Chapter 10.

Another way to use medication is to inject it directly into the muscles that are having involuntarily spasms. Medicines used in this manner stop the muscle spasms by blocking signals from the motor nerves that control those muscles. This type of nerve interruption is known as *chemodenervation* ("chemo" means "chemical," and "denervation" means "cutting or destroying nerves, or blocking their signals"). Formerly, solvent chemicals such as phenol were used for chemodenervation. Although such solvents still have useful applications, they have largely been replaced by botulinum toxin, a nerve toxin derived from bacteria. Botulinum toxin, marketed under trade names such as Botox, Myobloc, Dysport, and others, has become a mainstay of dystonia treatment. Botulinum toxin is discussed in Chapter 11.

In addition to chemodenervation, surgery can also be used to interrupt the nerve input to a muscle. This can be done by cutting specific nerves or even cutting the muscle itself. These techniques are usually applied to cervical dystonia. Surgery can also be done on the brain to interrupt the sending of abnormal signals from the basal ganglia, either by destroying a small area of brain tissue, or by implanting an electrical stimulator whose wire delivers disruptive signals to the basal ganglia. Use of this *deep brain stimulator* is primarily applied to generalized dystonias and some severe cases of cervical dystonia. It is discussed in Chapter 12.

3

Genetics of Dystonias

We have learned much more about how genetics influence our lives with the recent completion of the Human Genome Project, a worldwide endeavor to determine the location and functions of all human genes. We inherit half of our genes from each parent, and our unique combination of genes—a copy of which is contained in the chromosomes of nearly every cell of the body—acts as a blueprint to determine our physical characteristics.

Any particular characteristic determined by one or more genes is known as a trait. This includes some diseases. Just as we can inherit a blue eye trait from one parent and a dark hair trait from another, we can also inherit defective genes that can cause, or give us a tendency to develop, certain diseases, including dystonias. To date, 18 different genetic forms of dystonia have been identified and classified as DYT (short for dystonia) genes. Table 1 lists the different types of these genes and a brief description the type of dystonia. In some cases, this information is not known.

In general, the inherited forms of dystonia tend to start at a younger age and to involve the entire body. The way in which they are passed down within a family varies. Most dystonias are inherited in an *autosomal dominant* manner. This requires a little background explanation. You inherit two sets of genes: one set from your mother and one set from your father. For each type of gene, there is one *dominant* and one *recessive* variety. The dominant type is the form of the gene that is actually expressed (like having brown eyes). The recessive form is a form that is in the gene, but does not get expressed. For example, the brown eye trait is dominant to the blue eye trait. Therefore, when a child inherits a brown-eye trait from one parent and a blue-eye trait from the other parent, the child will (usually) end up with brown eyes. In the same manner, a defective gene that causes dystonia may be passed down dominantly in a family line,

Table 1   *Inherited Forms of Dystonias*

DYT Classification and Name	Gene	Type of Dystonia
DYT1 Oppenheim's dystonia	Torsin A 9q34	Generalized
DYT2	recessive	Generalized
DYT3 Lubag's dysonia	Xq13	Generalized
DYT4		Generalized
DYT5 Dopa-responsive dystonia	14q22 GTP cyclohydrolase I	Generalized
DYT6	8p11.21 THAP 1	Generalized
DYT7	18p	Focal – cervical dystonia
DYT8 Paroxysmal nonkinesogenic dyskinesia	2q31	Generalized
DYT9 Paroxysmal kinesogenic choreoathetosis With episodic ataxia and spasticity	1p	Generalized
DYT10 Paroxysmal kinesogenic dystonia	16p11.2-q12.1	Generalized
DYT11 Myoclonic dystonia	7q21; 11q23.1	Focal
DYT12 Rapid onset dystonia parkinsonism	19q12–113.2	Generalized
DYT13	1p36.32-p36.13	Generalized
DYT14 Dopa-responsive dystonia	Tyrosine hydroxylase	Generalized
DYT15 Myoclonic dysontia	18p11	Generalized
DYT16 Dystonia parkinsonism	2q31.3	Generalized
DYT17	20p11.2-q13.12	Generalized
DYT18 Paroxysmal exertion-induced dyskinesia	1p35-p31.3	Generalized

DYT, dystonia.

so that it only takes one parent passing down a defective gene for a child to have dystonia.

However, even though most dystonia-causing genes are dominant, they tend to have incomplete *penetrance*. This means the trait that they carry may not be fully expressed in the individual who inherits them; in other words, there may not be a one-to-one correspondence between inheriting the faulty gene and developing dystonia. Continuing with the eye-color analogy, since the trait for eye color also has reduced penetrance, not every child who inherits the brown-eye trait will have brown eyes. Some may have hazel or green eyes instead. More than one gene can be involved in producing a disorder. Sometimes one gene can give a person the tendency to develop dystonia. Such genes are called "susceptibility" genes because they don't cause the disease but instead put people at higher risk for developing it if they also have a second gene or other risk factor for dystonia. We have just begun to learn about these genes and how they work.

So you can see the genetic basis of dystonia is quite complex. We don't know every gene that can produce dystonia, so if you have a few family members with different forms of dystonia, there is a good chance that your dystonia could be one of the inherited types. There are genetic tests available to test for the more commonly inherited dystonias. But these genetic tests are usually very expensive and are not always paid for by insurance. Plus, there is always the question of what to do once the results of the test are known: not everyone who inherits the gene for dystonia will develop dystonia (because of incomplete penetrance), and currently there is no treatment for early dystonia that would influence the course of the disorder. The more commons forms of genetically inherited dystonia are as follows.

DYT-1, OPPENHEIM'S DYSTONIA

This form of inherited dystonia was first described a century ago by the German physician Hermann Oppenheim. It is found most commonly in the Ashkenazi Jewish population. It is caused by a mutation in the gene known as *DYT-1*, which resides, one each, on the ninth of the 23 pairs of chromosomes carried by humans. Oppenheim's dystonia generally develops in childhood, and the first area of the body affected is usually the foot or leg. It tends to progress to involve the entire body and is very disabling. It is inherited in an autosomal dominant fashion with variable penetrance. This means that, although the gene responsible for the disorder is passed down to the offspring 50 percent of the time, not everyone who inherits the gene develops the full-blown dystonia. Some may develop focal dystonias such as blepharospasm or cervical dystonia, and others will not have any dystonia. We think that there may be another gene or some other influence that determines whether a person with a defective *DYT-1* gene will develop generalized dystonia. Oppenheim's dystonia tends to respond well to implantation of an electronic deep-brain stimulator. A combination of medications can sometimes be helpful, including the anticholinergic medications trihexyphenidyl or benztropine and muscle relaxants, such as diazepam or lorazepam. These treatments will be discussed in Chapters 10 through 13.

DYT-5, DOPA-RESPONSIVE DYSTONIA

Dopa-responsive dystonia, labeled DYT-5, is also inherited in an autosomal dominant fashion with variable penetrance. It is caused by a mutation in the *GCH-1* gene on chromosome 14. It begins in childhood and most of the time starts in the foot or leg. The dystonia tends to spread and usually involves the entire body. One of the unique features of DYT-5 is that it tends to get worse over the course of the day. Sometimes people with this disorder develop features similar to those of Parkinson disease, including muscular rigidity and slowness in their movements.

Another unique feature is that the dystonia tends to improve dramatically with low doses of *levodopa*, a medication used to treat Parkinson disease. This improvement occurs because the gene defect that produces DYT-5 causes a deficiency of the brain chemical *dopamine*. Dopamine deficiency also occurs in Parkinson disease. Levodopa supplies dopamine to the brain, thus correcting the deficit. Levodopa is effective for both diseases.

Dopa-responsive dystonia is variable in penetrance, so not everyone who has inherited the gene will develop the full-blown dystonia. Some family members will develop focal dystonia such as blepharospasm or cervical dystonia; others will not develop dystonia at all. Even though DYT-5 represents only a small fraction of dystonia cases, we believe that because of this dramatic response to levodopa, almost all patients with any focal or generalized dystonia should be tried on at least a short course of the medication to gauge their response.

Another form of dopa-responsive dystonia is designated as DYT14. The gene defect responsible for it causes a deficiency in tyrosine hydroxylase, an enzyme that is important in the production of dopamine. When the level of the enzyme is deficient, the amount of dopamine produced is also deficient. This dystonic disorder is more severe than DYT-5 and begins in infancy. The most severely affected individuals do not survive.

4

Causes of Dystonias

Primary (idiopathic) dystonias arise "out of the blue" without an identifiable cause outside the nervous system. Some primary dystonias are associated with known genetic defects, as we discussed in Chapter 3, but in the majority of cases no specific genetic defect has been identified. Secondary dystonias are caused by another disease or external agent. These causes are discussed in more detail in this chapter. Most of these causative factors can result in dystonias that are focal (limited to one body part) or generalized over the whole body. Thus, they can produce almost any of the syndromes listed in Table 1 in Chapter 2.

MEDICATIONS

Medication side effects are the most common cause of acquired secondary dystonias. Most medications that produce dystonia have the pharmaceutical action of blocking the activity of the brain chemical *dopamine*. Such medications include antinausea drugs such as Compazine (prochlorperazine) or Reglan (metaclopramide). These dopamine-blocking medications are sometimes given intravenously to cancer patients, who may suffer severe nausea and vomiting as a side effect of chemotherapy. Large doses of antinausea medications given at any time may produce acute dystonia or dyskinesia in any body part or in the whole body. Such acute reactions are generally temporary and usually stop when the medicine is discontinued. Prolonged or permanent cases, termed *tardive dystonia* or *tardive dyskinesia,* discussed below in relation to similar medicines, are fortunately rare.

Acute dystonias can be reduced with doses of Benadryl (diphenhydramine) or Artane (trihexphenidyl). Temporary acute dyskinesia can also occur in some patients with advanced Parkinson's disease who require large doses of dopamine-enhancing medications.

Dystonia and dyskinesia can also develop as a permanent disorder after long-term use of dopamine-blocking medications. Certain psychiatric patients require long-term treatment with medications known as *neuroleptics* or *antipsychotics* in order to remain active and functional outside of a psychiatric institution. Chronic use of these medications may also result in the occurrence of late-onset, or *tardive*, dystonia or dyskinesia. The list of such medications is long, but it includes Haldol (haloperidol), Thorazine (thioridazine), Zyprexa (olanzapine), and Risperdal (risperidone). Since newer generation neuroleptics have a much lower tendency to produce such side effects, drug-induced movement disorders are becoming less common.

It is important to note that the most commonly used psychiatric medications are antidepressants such as Elavil (amitryptiline), Prozac (fluoxetine), Paxil (paroxetine), or Zoloft (sertraline), and many others. These medicines are not dopamine-blocking agents and are very rarely implicated in the development of movement disorders.

BRAIN DAMAGE

Brain damage suffered during fetal development in the womb or during infancy or early childhood may predispose an individual to develop dystonia later in life. Such early damage may be the result of complications during pregnancy or birth that cause oxygen deprivation. It can also be caused by fetal jaundice, in which toxins from the breakdown of blood cells and from liver dysfunction accumulate in the basal ganglia of the brain; or by an early brain infection (*encephalitis*) caused by bacteria, viruses, or certain parasites.

Any trauma causing respiratory or breathing failure in adulthood may result in brain damage and dystonia if the resulting oxygen deprivation, or *anoxia*, is severe enough to cause prolonged loss of consciousness or coma. Such anoxia may occur during a heart attack if rescuers are unable to resuscitate the victim quickly. Anoxia may also result from a drug overdose that depresses breathing. Such overdoses may occur accidentally during recreational drug abuse or a failed suicide attempt. Near-drowning or suffocation is another cause of anoxia. Anoxia has a predilection for harming components of the extrapyramidal system, including the basal ganglia.

A severe blow to the head that produces coma for a length of time may result in a number of neurologic deficits, including dystonia.

People who suffer brain damage from anoxia or trauma usually do not simply have dystonia alone. Such people almost always have memory problems, difficulty in understanding and communicating in verbal or written language, other cognitive deficits, incoordination of movements, or even paralysis of body parts in addition to dystonia. A single concussive blow to the head that only causes dizziness, or even transient loss of consciousness will not produce dystonia.

STROKE

A stroke occurs as a result of the plugging, or occlusion, of a brain artery, leading to the death of neurons and other brain cells in the territory supplied by that artery. Alternatively, a stroke may occur because of rupture and blood leakage from an artery. Occasionally, strokes that involve the basal ganglia or other parts of the extrapyramidal system will result in a dystonia. Only a small fraction of all strokes affect the extrapyramidal system in this way. A much larger percentage of strokes affect the primary pyramidal motor system, resulting in muscular weakness or paralysis in the affected body part. True muscle weakness of this type is not a feature of dystonia.

TOXINS

Medications that alter the activity of the brain chemical dopamine may produce a permanent tardive dystonia. These medications have been discussed above. Other environmental toxins are also known to produce movement disorders that can resemble dystonia. For example, the metallic element manganese has produced movement disorders among those who mine ore, and mercury or lead contamination from industrial sources can also cause movement disorder symptoms. Fortunately, with improved industrial safety practices, such cases have become much less common.

MEDICAL DISORDERS

Medical disorders that usually affect other parts of the body may produce dystonia or other movement disorders if the brain becomes involved. One such disorder is *systemic lupus erythmatosus,* also known as SLE, or just lupus. In this disorder, the immune system begins to attack normal body tissues, including those of blood vessels in the brain and the brain tissue itself. Other such medical conditions include Sydenham chorea, a later complication of rheumatic heart disease; Wilson disease, a complication of the body's inability to utilize the essential mineral copper; and some inborn problems with metabolizing certain nutrients. Some neurological diseases such as Huntington chorea and Parkinson disease may have dystonia among their symptoms.

Almost all of these medical conditions produce a variety of physical signs and symptoms that distinguish them from primary dystonia.

PHYSICAL INJURY

Physical injury deserves special discussion as a cause of cervical dystonia. Physical brain trauma that produces dystonia has been discussed above, and it is usually accompanied by a number of other neurologic impairments. What we discuss here is the onset of dystonia after *peripheral* trauma. Only a small fraction of all physical traumas result in development of dystonia. When dystonia occurs, it is most frequently in neck injury, producing cervical dystonia. This type of posttraumatic cervical dystonia is further discussed in Chapter 13. Limb and trunk dystonias can also occur after physical peripheral trauma, but these are much less common. The mechanism by which such injuries cause dystonia is not known.

5

Blepharospasm and Meige Syndrome

■

PATIENT PERSPECTIVE

I was born in Sweden, where I grew up and completed my training as a psychiatric nurse. After my husband and I retired in the mid-1990s, we decided to spend some years cruising on our boat in Mexican waters. In the early 90s, I started to have some discomfort in my eyes: blinking, dryness, and sometimes an inability to look upward. The latter problem actually led me to become lost while driving because I could not see the street signs. I visited my eye doctor, who treated me for dry eye. The problem persisted, and my doctor consulted with several colleagues about my condition. They could offer nothing but the dry eye diagnosis I already had, and the observation that I was getting older.

I was frequently uncomfortable in social situations or watching television, as my eyes would blink or close and I could not look up. Reading became difficult. When out walking, I would sometimes bump into things or people, once even walking into the side of a truck. I was wondering if I was crazy. I was able to do tasks only with a lot of focusing, but felt uncertain in the world. Later even swimming would become unbearably painful when water splashed in my eyes.

We made frequent trips to California for doctor's appointments. I was taking medication at night for sleep, and I noted that I was then able to read for several hours. That was a clue for me, which I later came to understand. These three years were very depressing, to the point where I was having suicidal thoughts.

One day another physician that I saw said the magical words, "I think you have a mild case of blepharospasm," and explained the nature of the disease. He went on to say that he knew a physician who was experienced at injecting Botox. I had tears running down my face as we exited the building. I wasn't crazy after all—there was a name and a treatment for my problem. I was overwhelmed with gratitude and wrote the doctor telling him so.

After just a small trial dose of Botox, I knew it was the answer. We returned from our cruising every three months to obtain treatment. There were not always good days, but my life had forever changed. I had hope. As time went by, I noticed that sleeping pills still had a beneficial effect, and that when I took an antihistamine I also sometimes felt relief from symptoms. That made me think that medications used for other movement disorders might also prove useful. I also suspected that I might have some additional dystonia. For those I would need a neurologist. Just at that time my UCLA doctor decided to move his practice out of state, so I wrote to the Benign Essential Blepharospasm Research Foundation (BEBRF) asking for neurologists in our area. Among others, I was given the name of a local neurologist and expert in movement disorders. He treated my blepharospasm with Botox and oral medication and has also treated me for spasmodic dysphonia.

A whole new life was ahead of me again. When running increased my blinking, I replaced it with Pilates exercises in a gym. I could still ski, and boating and fishing were not a problem. The wind and sun do not affect me as they do some people with blepharospasm, although I now try to protect my eyes more than I used to. Just recently, at the urging of my rehabilitation specialist, I have taken up the exercise of stand-up paddle boarding in order to help maintain my balance.

I think I am trying to live the words of Robert Louis Stevenson: "Life is not a matter of holding good cards, but of playing a poor hand well."

MEDICAL PERSPECTIVE

Blepharospasm is a rare dystonia affecting the muscles of the eye. The main symptom is uncontrollable squinting or closing of the eyelid. Milder forms of blepharospasm produce excessive blinking and more severe forms result in forced eye closure for prolonged periods of time. It can occur only in one eyelid, but it usually affects both eyes. Oftentimes, patients will raise their eyebrows to help keep their eyes open. This tends to produce wrinkles across the forehead, which can be a telltale sign of blepharospasm (Figure 1). Blepharospasm can interfere with vision, and can be disabling if the spasms are frequent or last long enough. As the patient above described, certain things can trigger the eyelid spasms.

Bright sunlight, wind, stress, and certain activities such as walking or running can trigger blepharospasm. On the other hand,

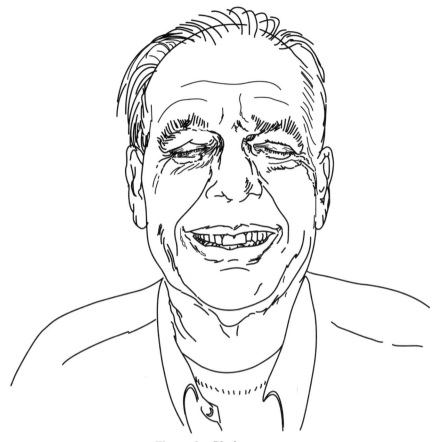

Figure 1 *Blepharospasm.*
Note the elevation of the eyebrows and wrinkling of the forehead in an attempt
to keep the eyes open.

performing activities such as humming, singing, talking, pinching the neck or touching the eyelids can sometimes relieve the symptoms of blepharospasm. Sudden forced closure of the eyelids while driving is dangerous. If severe enough, blepharospasm can produce functional blindness: patients who cannot keep their eyelids open cannot see.

Like other types of dystonia, the cause of blepharospasm is unknown. Blepharospasm tends to affect women more often than men, and it tends to start after age 50. Just as with other forms of dystonia, there may be a genetic factor involved. Secondary forms may occur following stroke, with certain drugs or drug withdrawal, or following injury to the eye area or surgery on the eyes. It is important to bring a list of all of medications to the doctor's visit, including medications one may have been taking when one first noted the blepharospasm and that have been discontinued.

PATIENT PERSPECTIVE

I have always had sensitivity to bright sunlight. Over the past two to three years I found that I could not walk outside without wearing sunglasses. My eyes would blink and close automatically. I even started wearing my sunglasses inside at work under the fluorescent lights.

My eyes would stay closed for a long time and I could not seem to open them without using my fingers. I stopped driving for fear of my eyes closing on me while I was on the road. Getting rides from friends and coworkers was difficult, but it was all I could do. I could no longer go shopping, and cleaning my house was difficult. I found that singing some of my favorite songs helped keep my eyes open, but you can't sing everywhere. After diagnosis and treatment with Botox injections, it became easier to keep my eyes open. They still close sometimes, but I no longer have to keep my eyes open with my fingers, and as an added bonus, the darkening of the skin around my eyes has become lighter.

A trial with artificial tears can help to differentiate blepharospasm from blinking caused by dry eye conditions. When dry eye is treated with artificial tears, patients no longer blink excessively or have eye closure spasms; this is not the case with blepharospasm.

Currently, the best treatment for blepharospasm is botulinum toxin injections into the *orbicularis oculi*, the disc-shaped muscle that encircles each eye socket. Botulinum toxin weakens this muscle and allows it to relax, reducing uncontrollable blinking and allowing patients to keep their eyes open more easily.

Although it is customary to have the treatment every three months, in many patients notice the toxin wears off sooner, and bothersome eye spasms return at 2 to 2.5 months. However, if a higher dose of toxin is used, drooping of the eyelid may result. Other side effects include bruising and dry eye. Some patients may report losing eyelashes.

MEIGE SYNDROME

PATIENT PERSPECTIVE

I was working in the school district when I first noted symptoms. I found it was difficult to talk and my speech sounded funny - my words would slur as if I were drunk. Sometimes my tongue would stick out of my mouth. This occurred for short periods of time at first. Eventually, the speech problem became constant. I found I was making faces when I tried to talk. My eyes would blink and close. I had trouble keeping my eyes open. My head began to shake. Food came out of my mouth when I tried to eat. It took several doctors and my own research into my condition before I would be diagnosed with Meige syndrome.

I was desperate—no one could understand me. I entered a research trial in which I received botulinum toxin injections in my neck for the head movements, and a wonderful thing happened: I went into remission. My voice sounded normal. My eyes stopped closing shut and my head stopped shaking. This occurred for about five years. Then one day I noticed my speech started to slur again. I used several tricks such as holding my neck or pushing along the side of my windpipe to help normalize my voice especially when talking on the phone. This helped for a while.

My speech fluctuates in and out from slurred to normal during the course of a conversation. My voice is worst when I am under stress. Phone calls are very stressful. I try not to talk unless I have to when my voice is bad. Relaxation techniques have helped me to cope. It is incredible, but when I go on vacation and am having fun, my voice sounds normal and I don't have to even think about it! I still have hope for another remission.

MEDICAL PERSPECTIVE

Sometimes blepharospasm is accompanied by dystonia of the facial muscles, pharynx muscles (muscles in the back of the throat that are involved in speech and swallowing), the tongue, and the vocal cords. When this occurs, it is called Meige syndrome. Sometimes the mouth is pulled to the side, the apples of the cheeks spasm, or there is a frowning appearance. When tongue movement or the pharyngeal muscles are involved, the speech sounds slurred, distorted and indistinct, similar to when a deaf person speaks. Tongue movement can affect chewing and swallowing in addition to speech.

Dystonia can also involve muscles of the jaws and mouth. This type of dystonia is called *oromandibular dystonia.* Symptoms can include difficulty opening the mouth, clenching or grinding of teeth, jaw spasms, sideways movement of the jaw, lip tightening or pursing, and abnormal movement of the tongue. The jaw may close or be forced open in oromandibular dystonia. Such involuntary postures may be intermittent or sustained. The grinding of the teeth can wear down tooth enamel. These symptoms can lead to jaw pain, difficulties eating and drinking, and sometimes difficulty speaking. Oromandibular dystonia can also be a feature of Meige syndrome.

Meige syndrome and oromandibular dystonia are also usually of unknown cause, and most of the time they occur without any precipitating injury. Genetic factors may play a role, as seen in other forms of dystonia. Oromandibular dystonia has been reported after dental procedures or jaw injury. Dental prosthetics can worsen symptoms of oromandibular dystonia. Temporomandibular joint syndrome (TMJ) can occur as a result of oromandibular dystonia. Stress tends to worsen or bring on symptoms of Meige syndrome and oromandibular dystonia. Some patients find that humming or singing improves their symptoms. Patients who suffer from grinding of the teeth report that chewing a toothpick relieves their symptoms. The facial grimacing may be annoying and interfere with social and professional activities. In such cases, it is advisable to let people know about your condition and that you are not grimacing at them.

Remission of symptoms occurs rarely. A remission generally occurs spontaneously regardless of treatment or activity; however, symptoms tend to reoccur after a period of time. For the most part, these disorders are lifelong.

The facial grimacing can be treated with botulinum toxin. Extensive treatment should be avoided as the face could become droopy. Teeth grinding can be treated by injecting boutulinum toxin into the muscle responsible for the grinding. The result here is quite good. However, treatment of dystonia involving the tongue is tricky. The tongue's three-dimensional and finely synchronized movements are difficult to restore by botulinum toxin injection. The treatment should be done only by the most experienced movement specialists.

6

Spasmodic Dysphonia

■

PATIENT PERSPECTIVE

It seemed like it happened overnight. In meetings, giving speeches, talking in front of groups had become quite difficult. My voice didn't seem to respond effortlessly, as it once had. It was like trying to talk while someone was gripping my throat. It felt like a misfiring piston.

As the CEO of a large insurance company where communication was the lifeblood of my success, that created some real problems. I even began to question whether I could continue to be effective at my job and considered early retirement. Not knowing what to do, I went to see an ear, nose, and throat doctor. He seemed perplexed, but sent me to a speech therapist. After 3 months with no results, I was feeling rather hopeless and worried. I was not sure where next to turn.

Hearing me struggle at a speaking engagement, my boss, the chairman of the company, said, "We've got to find out what's going on with your voice." He asked our company chief medical officer to do some research. Several weeks later he called and asked the question that started me on this journey: "Have any of the doctors mentioned spasmodic dysphonia?" I responded, "Not a one!"

MEDICAL PERSPECTIVE

Spasmodic dysphonia is caused by involuntary movements of the muscles of the voice box. It is believed to affect less than 200,000 people in the United States. The symptoms generally start when individuals are between 30 and 50 years of age, and the disorder more often affects women than men. The symptoms can be so minor as to be barely noticeable, or can be severe enough to be socially or professionally disabling.

It is important to distinguish spasmodic dysphonia from other conditions that cause hoarseness of the voice, like laryngitis, muscle tension disorder, chronic reflux of stomach acid, and other types of throat irritation. Most such disorders do not produce restriction or change in airflow.

There are different types of spasmodic dysphonia. The muscles of the voice box can be affected by being pulled together or being pulled apart.

In *ad*ductor spasmodic dysphonia, the muscles of the voice box are pulled together and the voice has a strained, disconnected quality. Patients have difficulty speaking loudly. In its severe form, this type of spasmodic dysphonia can cause irregular, choppy speech, with brief periods of silence when the muscle contractions interrupt air flow. Vowels are often split in pronunciation. Speaking on the phone is especially difficult. The patients feel like their voices are choked off. They can, however, scream or laugh aloud without spasm. They also have no spasm when whispering or singing in high pitch. Stress commonly worsens speech symptoms, and the voices tend to improve when the patients are emotional. These features not uncommonly lead to the misdiagnosis of psychological disorder.

Adductor spasmodic dysphonia is the most common form. In the less common *ab*ductor spasmodic dysphonia, the muscles of the voice box are pulled apart, and the voice has a breathy, whispery quality and is not choppy. Some patients have both types of spasmodic dysphonia, which creates a mixture of symptoms.

Spasmodic dysphonia can occur by itself, or in combination with other dystonias like those involving the face and neck. The body parts that are most commonly involved are the lower face, jaw, tongue, and neck. For these patients, on average the duration before spreading is 7.3 years. Spasmodic dysphonia may coexist with vocal tremor.

■

PATIENT PERSPECTIVE

I started singing in school plays at the age of nine, and continued into high school by taking four years of music/choir and singing in the church choir. As an adult, I continued to participate in church choir, Christmas, and Easter programs. I became involved in community theater and part of the staged crowd in the musicals. Then in 1988, at age 48, my singing voice began to leave me and became very raspy and strangulated. I was no longer able to sing and participate in what I had loved to do most of my life.

Along came botulinum toxin and my voice was on the soft side for about four weeks. I would sing in a lower volume until my voice got stronger, then I would have a better range to sing the harmony part in the choir with my alto voice. I have continued in my church choir from the beginning of my strangulated voice until this day.

Interestingly, patients who are singers may develop a dysphonia primarily in their singing voice, with the symptoms abating when they use normal conversational speech. However, when the condition is severe, conversational speech is involved as well. Some patients note improvement if they alter their pitch. When conversational speech is affected, they can communicate easier by whispering. This is understandable, as during whispering, the dystonic vocal cords are not being used.

PATIENT PERSPECTIVE

Twenty years ago I noticed that in cold weather breathing in brought a certain burning sensation to my throat. I dismissed it as something that just happened. When walking with friends they commented on my difficulty breathing, and I dismissed it as they were in better physical shape than I was in; and I was an artist, not an athlete.

In art classes people who worked next to me commented on the way I was breathing, and asked me whether or not I had asthma, or if I was getting a cold, or if I was generally stressed out. I felt normal and ignored it, thinking that I was just working hard and concentrating as hard as I could. To me, my breathing was normal, and I could never understand what they were talking about.

I used to derive a great deal of pleasure singing when I was a young girl, but noticed that I could no longer sing through a complete phrase. Even then, I dismissed it as being out of practice and having no professional training. I had heard about singers losing their voices and told myself the same thing was happening to me. I noticed that I had feelings of not being able to breathe comfortably, but dismissed it as anxiety.

One day I listened to the playback of my recording for my answering machine and I could not believe the sound of my voice. I noticed that I took a very deep breath before speaking and was only able to say a few words before I needed another breath. I was shocked by the quality of my voice.

Then my husband and I were videotaped and I watched myself, wondering who this person was—this person whose head kept nodding up and down. I knew that something was wrong and that I should seek help.

When I first went to a doctor, he blocked a nerve in my throat and asked me to speak. For thirty seconds I heard the voice I had as a teenager.

In some patients with spasmodic dysphonia, the symptoms cause shortness of breath due to the spasm of the laryngeal muscles, like in this patient. At times, to overcome the spasms, she would unknowingly take a deep breath before speaking and reflexively try to relax the spasm, or would instinctively soften her voice before speaking. Watching a videotape of herself caused her to realize that all these subconcious actions were actually responses to the symptoms of spasmodic dysphonia. She had accepted taking deep breaths as something normal and necessary in order to speak. In some patients, the spasmodic dysphonia is part of the Meige syndrome or of cervical dystonia, but the symptoms in the neck or eyes are milder and occur only intermittently. In this case, her head nodding was a symptom of cervical dystonia.

As seen in this case, blocking the nerve on one side of the vocal cords by injecting a local anesthetic can relax the spasm, allowing temporary improvement for the duration of the block. This nerve block could be used to confirm spasmodic dysphonia before exposing the patient to a longer effect of botulinum toxin.

PATIENT PERSPECTIVE

After I was diagnosed with spasmodic dysphonia, I went to a larger hospital out of state. After a few tests, they told me that I indeed had spasmodic dysphonia and needed to start treatment with Botox. Botox! I'm thinking, "That's the new trendy treatment for wrinkles. How in the world is that going to help me?" A few days later, I was in the doctor's office thinking that at the very least I'd have wrinkle-free vocal cords!

Four days after my first injection, I could barely whisper. Terrified that I'd permanently lost my voice, I called the doctor and whispered, "You'd better hope this works!" It did.

As luck or fate would have it, this rare disease was ironically shared by one of my assistants, who had been seeing another doctor and gave me his name. Little did I know at the time that I was about to see one of the most renowned experts in spasmodic dysphonia. It was then that my life began to change. The doctor consulted with me about options, explained thoroughly the nature of my affliction, and recommended alternating injections in one cord at a time. The results have made for a much shorter recovery time, much better voice quality, and much less stress about my voice response. It has allowed me to do what I do best—communicate with confidence.

They say you don't appreciate something until it's gone. Most people don't even think about talking, they just do it (sometimes too much!). While I do still think about it, now I think about it far less.

Historically, spasmodic dysphonia was thought to be psychological or traumatic in origin. The first organic approach was the surgery by Dr. Herbert Dedo of San Francisco, California, who, by cutting the nerve that supplied the vocal cord on one side, paralyzed that cord and prevented it from pulling together with the opposite side. Dr. Dedo's nerve surgeries were a bold solution at a time when his colleagues still advocated psychotherapy as the mainstay of treatment. This surgery has outstanding initial results, but symptoms may later return due to the enlargement of the opposite vocal cord, which begins to overlap the weakened operated side.

Although it responds poorly to oral medications, spasmodic dysphonia does respond well to injections of botulinum toxin into the laryngeal muscles. The effectiveness of botulinum toxin was first reported by Dr. Andrew Blitzer. Dr. Daniel Truong established botulinum toxin as the treatment of first choice for spasmodic dysphonia with the publication of a double blind study in which the effectiveness of botulinum toxin injection was proven in comparison with a placebo injection of salt water.

In comparison with the "all or nothing" results of nerve-cutting surgery, botulinum toxin injections allow adjustment of the dose to achieve graded degrees of vocal cord muscle weakening. Additionally, undesirable outcomes from surgery can be permanent, whereas such results from botulinum toxin will wear off over time. For instance, patients may have a short period of breathiness of the voice after injections, but this soon subsides and the voice normalizes. Breathiness occurs more often in female patients and the elderly. Breathiness is caused by too frequent opening of the windpipe. In this case, alternating injections limited to only one vocal cord at a time could be considered.

Although the injection would seem a little scary, it is quite straightforward and can be done quickly in experienced hands. Although side effects include breathiness, choking, and swallowing difficulty, these side effects are often short lived and mild.

7

Writer's Cramp and Occupational Dystonias

PATIENT PERSPECTIVE

I am a 40-year-old male and a finance director for a major health care company. I started to experience tremors in my dominant hand at the age of 15. The tremors would inexplicably originate from my forearms up to my palm and fingers.

Through university (age 21), the tremors became more apparent, and I began to augment my writing style by gripping the pen and holding the paper close to my body so more pressure could be placed on paper and pen.

By the time I started working (age 23), I had to modify how I wrote by using my thumb and forefinger to hold the pen completely vertical, which in time caused a lot of strain to my finger joint and knuckle.

By age 28, I decided to enter business school for an MBA. At this point I couldn't write an essay longer than a page before my right hand began to ache. Through sheer brute force, I began to teach myself to be ambidextrous. I could only write print, not hand cursive, with my left hand, but it at least got me through essays beyond a few pages. I graduated 2 years later and, unbelievably, tremors emerged in my left hand and began to increase quickly. I entered the work force, and luckily most of the work I dealt with was on a computer, using a keyboard and mouse. Clicking a button or typing with ten fingers did not appear to aggravate my handwriting... at least I didn't attribute it as much. Handwriting was often relegated to taking short notes at meetings and I was able to get by.

At this point (age 32), I reverted to using my right hand since the left was too unstable. Writing with my right again meant writing in an extremely contorted way. People would ask me about my writing, which made me self-conscious, but I did what I could and typed letters anytime I had to do long reports or take formal notes in a meeting. I guess I made the best of what I had.

MEDICAL PERSPECTIVE

Writer's cramp (WC) is a focal dystonia that usually begins in the dominant hand (the one used for writing). It is most often idiopathic and involves involuntary contraction of the hand, wrist, or forearm muscles, forcing these parts into abnormal postures while writing with pen or pencil. The pen may be gripped too tightly, or released and dropped, or held at an odd angle. The writing may be stretched upward, be otherwise distorted, or be poorly legible.

In the early stages, the cramps may happen only after the patient has been writing for a while—a page or more. Muscle aching and pain may develop shortly after starting to write. The development of pain usually does not show a relationship with the severity of writing impairment. The severity of pain is, however, associated with disability. The duration from starting to write until the pain appears shortens with time. Later in the course of the disorder, cramps may happen after only one sentence. It may even become difficult for a patient to sign name. Depending on how much writing is required by a patient's job, this can present significant problems.

WC may be classified as simple or complex. In simple WC, only the writing activities are affected. Other activities such as buttoning of clothes, handling fork and knives, etc. are unimpaired. In contrast, patients with complex WC (also called dystonic writer's cramp), have difficulty in these tasks as well. The initial simple WC can develop into complex WC when the condition is worsened by the continued use of the hand used for writing. WC is often associated with other dystonias, most commonly cervical dystonia and oromandibular dystonia.

WCs are divided into five different subtypes for treatment purposes: in the so-called "focal flexor subtype," (Figure 1) one or two fingers curl inward with writing activity. In the "generalized flexor subtype," both the fingers and the hand have the tendency to curl up (Figure 2), and aching and pain occur either on the palm or on the forearm. In the "focal extensor subtype," only one or two muscles that extend the fingers are involved (Figure 3). In the "generalized extensor subtype," the hand also extends (Figure 4), although different extensor muscles may be involved. In either extensor subtype, the patient will intermittently drop the pen due to involuntary finger extension. The patient may try to overcome this by flexing the

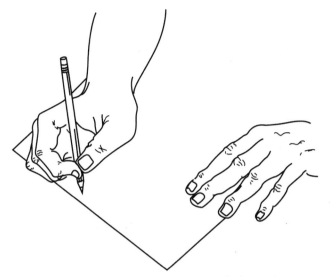

Figure 1 *Focal flexor subtype of writer's cramp.*

Source: From Das PD, Truong DD, Hallett M. Treatment of focal hand dystonia. In Truong DD, Dressler D, Hallet M, eds. Manual of Botulinum Toxin Therapy. New York: Cambridge University Press; 2009.

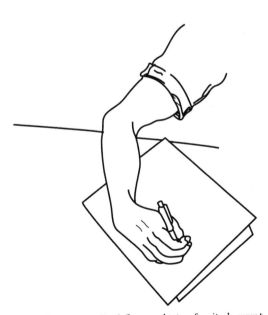

Figure 2 *Generalized flexor subtype of writer's cramp.*

Source: From Das PD, Truong DD, Hallett M. Treatment of focal hand dystonia. In Truong DD, Dressler D, Hallet M, eds. Manual of Botulinum Toxin Therapy. New York: Cambridge University Press; 2009.

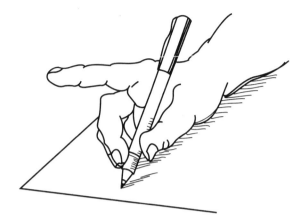

Figure 3   *Focal extensor subtype of writer's cramp.*

Source: From Das PD, Truong DD, Hallett M. Treatment of focal hand dystonia. In Truong DD, Dressler D, Hallet M, eds. Manual of Botulinum Toxin Therapy. New York: Cambridge University Press; 2009.

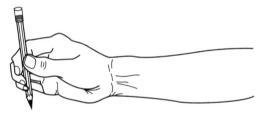

Figure 4   *Generalized extensor subtype of writer's cramp.*

Source: From Das PD, Truong DD, Hallett M. Treatment of focal hand dystonia. In Truong DD, Dressler D, Hallet M, eds. Manual of Botulinum Toxin Therapy. New York: Cambridge University Press; 2009.

fingers to hold the pen. Lastly, in the "arm abduction subtype," the arm moves away during attempted writing (Figure 5).

■

Patient Perspective

It was 1980, and I was madly trying to get my PhD thesis wrapped up. I was brimming over with excitement at completing it before I reached the age of 28. I had already set my short-term, intermediate, and long-term goals, with many targets to be completed before my 40th birthday. It was a long list of ambitious accomplishments, and little did I know that all my excitement was about to come to a rude end, probably for life.

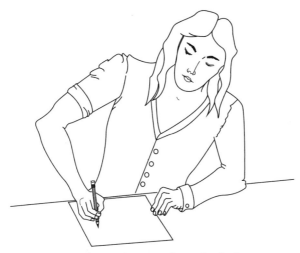

Figure 5   *Arm abduction subtype of writer's cramp.*

Source: From Das PD, Truong DD, Hallett M. Treatment of focal hand dystonia. In Truong DD, Dressler D, Hallet M, eds. Manual of Botulinum Toxin Therapy. New York: Cambridge University Press; 2009.

In June of 1980 I did not have the luxury of a computer or electronic type-writer, so I had to use the only instrument available: my hand. While writing my thesis, I noticed that I was experiencing some soreness from my right shoulder all the way down my arm to my fingers. Since getting my thesis completed was my only priority, I didn't pay much attention to the soreness until it got to a point where I had to go to the campus infirmary. I continued to write in pain as I was preparing the defense for my thesis.

As the problem with my arm worsened, I was frantically exploring names of doctors, their specialties, and whether or not anything could be done to get me out of this misery. I had reached the point where I could not write or do anything else requiring the use of my hands. This was the frightening part, and being right-handed made the situation worse. Twenty-eight sessions of chiropractic spinal manipulation and 300 acupuncture sessions brought me nowhere. Finally, a neurologist advised me to completely stop using my right hand for writing.

For the next year, I kept myself busy practicing to write with my left hand and trying to limit the use of my right hand. Slowly, I completely switched my writing from right to left. After many neurologists, I finally consulted a movement disorder specialist (not a self-appointed movement disorder expert). I was treated with Botox injections into my right arm. The first three times I didn't feel any difference; but very soon I started to feel much better. I continued the therapy and was confident that I was on the road to a new lease on life. It has been almost 15 years since I first got the treatment, and I have continued it on a regular basis to date.

Sometimes, patients adapt to WC by switching to writing with the opposite, non-dominant, hand. Unfortunately, WC tends to develop in the non-dominant hand as well in about 50% of the patients. About half of patients develop "mirror dystonia" (i.e., dystonic muscle activity) when they are writing with the opposite hand. Symptoms get worse in people who try to keep writing, and eventually other activities such as shaving, using utensils, and brushing teeth may become impaired. In extreme cases, the arm may assume the posture whenever the patient wants to use the hand.

■

PATIENT PERSPECTIVE

I was a successful flutist for over 10 years in Southern California. In the summer of 1988, I began playing a show that ran seven nights a week for 2 months. After playing so many consecutive nights, I began experiencing a new sensation in my left hand. At first, all I noticed was a "glitch" in a couple of my fingers not lifting all the time. There was no pain, but subtle problems with technique began to occur—problems I'd never had before. Musical passages and scales that had been easy before now became cumbersome and difficult.

My first reaction was to practice more, but the more I practiced, the worse the problem became. I noticed my left hand would cramp severely after playing just a short time, and within a few months, the only way I could play at all was to allow the hand to cramp and play on my knuckles. I tried using rubber bands to straighten the fingers and allow some movement, but this was frustrating and did little to help.

During the fall of 1988, most doctors I saw thought I was overusing my hand. This was diagnosed as the crux of my problem until I finally was referred to a neurologist. Instead of trying to explain my problem to the neurologist, I pulled out my flute and played a Mozart concerto for him. After a few bars, my left hand cramped, just as it always did. This doctor had worked with musicians on the East Coast, and knew immediately what was wrong. He presented me with the diagnosis of focal dystonia. He told me that in a few cases, after a year of rest, some or all of my technique could return without cramping, but the odds of that happening were slim and most musicians stop playing completely.

I tried taking a few months off, but had to continue playing for both financial and emotional reasons. I played with rubber bands twisted around my fingers to help the movement as best I could. I found that playing piccolo was easier than flute, due to the different positioning of the fingers of the left hand, and fortunately was able to continue to free-lance, although it was frustrating. Because I was fighting the cramping, my hand, arm, and shoulder became very painful. A month before I was to return for a follow-up visit with my neurologist, I read an article in the LA Times about a physician, "The Miracle Worker", and the methods he performed with dystonia and spasmodic torticollis patients using botulinum toxin injections directly into affected muscles.

I saw this movement disorder specialist for the first time in early 1990. At the time, I was preparing for a recital at the college where I was teaching and was having such a difficult time playing I considered canceling the recital. He injected my hand and wrist muscles on a Friday and warned that they would not have any effect for about 2 days, but that didn't stop me from trying to play immediately. All day Friday and Saturday there was no change, but on Sunday evening, I picked up the flute and played as I hadn't in years. The concerto I'd been working on for my recital, which had been so difficult and labored, was suddenly easy to play, and I couldn't stop practicing. The injections had worked, and I was able to perform without pain or cramping. It was difficult for me to button up my clothes, due to the weakness in the fingers, but that was a small price to pay for having my music career back.

I've been treated for over 19 years, and am still successfully performing. The injections don't always have the same effect—some injections work better than others—but I am grateful to be able to perform.

MEDICAL PERSPECTIVE

Occupational dystonias are also a type of focal dystonia. They occur when an individual has to perform with their hands during work, for example, in musicians who play instruments that require complicated finger movements as in the case above, or in people who have jobs such as assembly work that require repetitive hand motions.

Patients notice spasm and pain a short time after they start playing the instrument or performing the particular task. Their fingers feel glued together and heavy. They struggle to perform. The hand

and fingers assume abnormal postures, making a smooth performance difficult. The pain may intensify, necessitating a period of rest before the person can resume. Unfortunately, this is not always possible, such as during a musical performance. Initially, symptoms are present only during the causative activity, later they will also be present without the activity.

These types of dystonias do not respond well to most available treatments. Injections with botulinum toxin may help individuals to continue the necessary activities, but do not affect the cause of the symptoms in the brain. Even with botulinum toxin the results are limited, especially with musicians. A perfect dexterity or perfect handling of instruments is seldom achieved.

In musicians, even a slight weakness or incoordination may result in degradation of the performance. Few are able to continue their profession unimpeded. Some try to switch hands, but soon same problem occurs in the other hand.

The best advice is to scale down the amount of practice. The determined patient will, however, do the opposite. They try even harder to overcome and practice even more. Alternating with another instrument is also advisable as it changes the pattern of repetitive overuse, as it did for our patient above. However, switching to another instrument fully is not an answer either. Soon it will occur with this instrument as well.

8

Paroxysmal Dystonias

PATIENT PERSPECTIVE

For as long as I can remember, I have always moved funny. I mean, when I get up out of a chair or I start to run or walk, my body makes a funny movement. My hand and arm will flex or jerk. My foot will turn in or my body will twist. This happens for a short period of time and then goes away. When I was involved in track in high school, these movements interfered with my stride. Sometimes I can feel them coming on, but most of the time I just try to cover them up. I have taken seizure medications for this since I was a teenager. The medications tend to reduce the movements, but sometimes they still occur, and side effects from the medications make me feel foggy and I have difficulty concentrating. This has become more of a problem now that I am pursuing a career in acting. I have had to retake scenes several times because of these movements, which tend to be worse when I am under stress. Typically for my trade, I am also employed as a waiter, and have spilled drinks when moving around. I feel like a freak. I am hopeful that one day the perfect medication will exist; I won't have any more abnormal movements, and still feel normal.

MEDICAL PERSPECTIVE

The paroxysmal dystonias are composed of four types: *paroxysmal kinesogenic dyskinesia, paroxysmal nonkinesogenic dyskinesia, paroxysmal exertion induced dyskinesia,* and *paroxysmal hypnogenic dyskinesia.*

The term "paroxysmal" refers to something that happens episodically as opposed to occurring continuously. The term dyskinesia refers to movements that can be dystonic with twisting and sustained postures; choreiform, which are movements with a dancelike quality; or ballistic, which are larger more exaggerated movements, such as swinging the arm up and down. These conditions produce any of the above types of movements or, more usually, a combination of these movements.

Paroxysmal kinesogenic dyskinesia (PKD) refers to the onset of the dyskinesia with movement. This is illustrated in the patient's perspective above. The movement tends to be dystonic, but a combination of choreiform or ballistic (flinging) movements can be seen. The abnormal *involuntary* movements tend to occur after the patient makes a sudden *voluntary* momement, such as the starting of a foot race, or may begin after a period of rest. The attacks are brief, lasting seconds to minutes, and can occur on one side of the body or even be localized to one limb. PKD is often inherited in an autosomal dominant fashion and tends to occur more often in males. It usually begins in childhood and the average age that the condition first occurs ranges from 5 to 15 years of age. This disorder is treated differently than other forms of dystonia as it tends to respond to seizure medications. Effective seizure medications include phenytoin, valproic acid, carbamazepine and acetazolamide.

Paroxysmal nonkinesogenic dystonia (PKND) has its attacks of dyskinesia occuring without movement. It can be inherited in an autosomal dominant fashion and also occurs more frequently in males. It can start during childhood up through the twenties. Attacks tend to be of longer duration than in PKD, lasting minutes to hours. Movement does not precipitate an attack. Alcohol, caffeine, emotional excitement, or stress can trigger PKND. Attacks can be relieved by sleep. Avoidance of triggers can be helpful. Treatment of PKND is with medications such as clonazepam, anticholinergics, and sometimes antiepileptic agents.

Exercise may provoke attacks of dystonia in paroxysmal exertional induced dyskinesia (PED). PED is also inherited in an autosomal dominant fashion. The attacks appear similar as in PKD, however they occur more frequently in the legs. The attacks can occur in the arms if there is exercise limited to the upper extremities. Age of onset can range from childhood to early twenties. Avoidance of prolonged exercise and sometimes medications such as levodopa can be effective.

Similar attacks of dyskinesias occurring during sleep character-ize paroxysmal hypnognic dyskinesia (PHD). These movements last seconds to minutes. Sometimes these attacks can occur during the daytime as well. Some of these attacks are thought to be seizures affecting the frontal lobes of the brain. A treatment with seizure medications tends to be effective.

9

Generalized Dystonias

■

PATIENT PERSPECTIVE

I can remember when my daughter Kris was in about the fourth grade that her teachers would comment on how tightly she gripped her pencil with her right hand when she wrote. It was so tight, they said, that the pencil would leave its imprint on her fingers. Kris would tell me her hand was tired from writing. I would accuse her of being lazy and say that she needed to get back to her homework. I feel guilty about that now.

When Kris was in junior high, she came home excited one day because she said she found out she could write easier with her left hand. I feel guilty about that too, feeling I forced her to become a right handed person when she should have been left dominant.

In high school, when her hand tremors and control worsened, we realized Kris had a medical problem, and she was diagnosed as having a focal dystonia, in particular, writer's cramp.

Kris was treated for several months with Botox injections. These helped alleviate her symptoms, but she grew immune to the effects of that particular strain of botulinum toxin and had to quit the injections. Unfortunately her condition continued to worsen with time. She developed symptoms in the neck and trunk. At meals food would fling from her utensils because she couldn't control her hand movements. When she spoke, you could hear the effects on her voice. She had to take naps because her body was tired from fighting itself. Little did I know it was worse than that. When she would bathe and shave her legs, the water would become red from the nicks and cuts she would get because she couldn't hold the razor steady.

MEDICAL PERSPECTIVE

Generalized dystonia is a rare condition that often starts as a localized dystonia, but progresses over months or years to include the spine, trunk, and limbs. Generalized dystonia is a disabling condition that can interfere with the ability to keep a job, care for oneself independently, and in extreme cases, to walk. This is an inherited condition that often starts in childhood. Some people with generalized dystonia have a specific gene abnormality that is passed to their children, but not everyone who has this version of the gene gets symptoms.

The symptoms usually begin in a pre-adolescent or teenage individual who is otherwise healthy. The symptoms may start as a foot that turns in or twists during walking, but straightens out when walking quickly or running, and relaxes at rest. Alternatively, the individual's arm may either twist or straighten out when doing things like dressing, eating, writing, or playing an instrument.

At first, the involuntary movement or muscle spasm will only partly interfere with the activity that brings it on (like walking in the case of the turned foot, or dressing in the case of the twisted arm), and it will stop when the activity is over. However, over months or years, the symptoms progress to include spasms during additional activities using the same body part, or in a "mirror" fashion when the limb on the opposite side is used, and may continue when at rest. Eventually, the dystonia may then completely interfere with the ability to perform the activity. It may at this point take a fixed posture.

PATIENT PERSPECTIVE

In 1982, at the age of 10, I first noticed my left foot turning in. I went from doctor to doctor for almost 2 years before I was diagnosed. I was told everything: I had this and that. I had several surgeries on my foot. I tried all kinds of medications and nothing was working at all. I was beginning to give up hope. I thought that they should cut off my foot and gave me an artificial one.

Finally, I was diagnosed as having dystonia musculorum deformans (another name for generalized dystonia). I was given Tegretol and Valium and then sent home. I had some orthopedic surgery on muscles in my left foot, and this worked for several years. I was walking normally again. Two years later, all my symptoms were back and worse than they had ever been. I was immediately put on Sinemet and Parsidol. I stayed on Tegretol and was also taking Artane, and I never felt so horrible in my life.

My symptoms progressed. After a few years, my back would arch back-ward. My hips became lopsided. Slowly my neck began turning to one side. I tried several new medications. Some worked, some didn't. I even received Botox in my back because my trunk was spasming out of control. I went from one type of botulinum toxin to another, switching back and forth for about a year until I built up resistance to both types, and they no longer worked. I then quit botulinum toxin injection. I remember one time that my spasms were so bad that the needle broke off in my back muscle. By the year 2001, I could barely walk. I used a cane. I tried a long staff to hold myself up—anything to stay off of a wheelchair.

As the disease progresses, symptoms start to affect another limb, usually the opposite arm or leg. Over time, more and more muscles become affected in the limbs, and the dystonia progresses towards the torso. The dystonia in the torso causes abnormal posture and affects the ankle or wrist, then knee or elbow, hip or shoulder, and eventually the muscles of the torso and spine. Involvement of spinal muscles may cause pain from the lower back to the neck. In many cases, uncontrollable bending or twisting of the neck in one or more directions makes it impossible to look straight ahead (Figure 1).

Symptoms may creep into muscles of the face and mouth, produc-ing uncontrollable grimacing facial expressions and slurred speech. The body begins to twist and gyrate more persistently throughout the day, interfering more and more with all activities including work, school, play, eating, dressing, and bathing. A cane or walker may be required, or even a wheelchair if walking becomes too difficult or balance is affected.

The dystonic movements are generally of slow or medium speed, with a writhing and twisting quality. Sometimes the movements are faster or jerkier, occasionally creating violent flinging motions. In the worst cases, the torso, neck, and all the limbs are in continu-ous motion during waking hours, and the individual is constantly in a contorted posture, becoming physically incapacitated, unable to walk or even sit.

In almost all cases, the dystonic muscle spasms get better when the person is at rest and go away completely during sleep. Unless there are other complicating factors, the mind, including all cogni-tive abilities, is unaffected. The person is able to see, hear, feel, com-municate, understand and reason without limitation. Even among

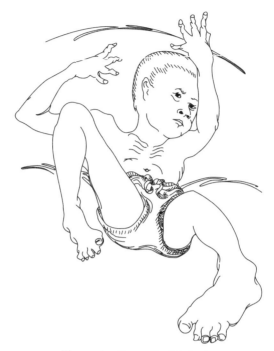

Figure 1   *Generalized dystonia.*

the physically disabled, the disorder is not fatal, and lifespan is not affected.

The scenario described above is a mixture of the natural history of generalized dystonia experienced among the majority of patients and will not be accurate for any one individual. The age of onset may vary, although starting before five or after the mid-twenties is rare. Not all patients will progress to the incapacity of the worst case. Generally, the disorder reaches its worst progression within the first 5 years of onset and then remains stable.

Various factors may predict the eventual degree of spread and severity. For dystonia beginning in any body part, the earlier the age of onset, the more likely it is to progress to a generalized syndrome. Dystonia starting in the upper limbs or neck, as is more common among adults, is less likely to spread elsewhere, whereas onset in the lower limbs, as is more common among children, portends future advancement to generalized dystonia. The wrists and hands are often spared from involvement in generalized dystonia.

There are various types of generalized dystonia, some with iden-tifiable causes and some without. There have been a number of schemes to classify and name the various types. One way has been to simply classify them by age of onset: early being 0 to 12 years, ado-lescent being 13 to 20 years, and adult onset being after 20 years of age. Another method is to classify them as *primary*, that is, a dystonia arising by itself, perhaps from a genetic defect, but usually without identifiable cause; and *secondary*, that is, occurring as an effect of some other disease, injury, medication, toxin, or condition affect-ing certain parts of the brain, particularly the basal ganglia. These causative factors have been discussed in Chapter 4.

TREATMENT OF GENERALIZED DYSTONIA

Medicines used to treat dystonia can be divided into two categories: those that are ingested orally and exert their action diffusely all over the body, and those that are injected locally and act only in targeted muscles. Among oral medications, the use of the Parkinson disease drug levodopa has already been discussed and is extremely effec-tive for the specific type of dystonia labeled as dopamine-responsive. Unfortunately, this accounts for only a small fraction of all dysto-nia cases. The vast majority of cases are not dopamine-responsive and other medications work only marginally well for them. In a few cases, especially those with spastic limbs and brisk tendon-jerk reflexes, muscle relaxant medications such as baclofen can be of use. Pharmacological treatment is described in detail in Chapter 10.

Another medicinal approach in generalized dystonia is the delivery of medication directly into the fluid surrounding the spi-nal cord. This is accomplished by means of an *intrathecal pump*. This battery-operated electronic device is implanted under the skin of the abdomen. A thin tubular catheter runs from the pump into the spinal canal, where it penetrates the lining around the spinal cord and drips medication directly into the spinal fluid. This pump and its attached catheter are completely internal; only the outline of the stopwatch-sized pump is visible under the skin of the lower abdo-men. A doctor programs the dose delivery rate of the pump, as well as refills the pump when necessary by injecting medication through the skin and into the pump reservoir using an ordinary syringe and needle. The two medications most commonly used in intrathecal pumps are baclofen, the antispasticity medication, and morphine or one of its related drugs, used for pain control.

Unfortunately, botulinum toxin, which is effective for focal or localized dystonias, is difficult to apply to generalized dystonia. Too many muscles are involved here, many of them too large and powerful to be treated with the toxin. It may have limited application in generalized dystonia if limited to a particular body part that is most troublesome.

One surgical option is for the surgeon to insert a probe to destroy a small part of the basal ganglia, either in a part called the *globus pallidus* (pallidotomy) or in a part called the *thalamus* (thalamotomy). This procedure creates, in effect, a small stroke that may disrupt abnormal brain signals causing dystonia. The surgery is technically difficult, requiring MRI guidance to ensure precision placement of the destructive lesion. This approach carries a small risk of stroke, and the results are more or less permanent and difficult to change. The latest, and increasingly most popular, surgical option is deep brain stimulation (DBS), which is covered in Chapter 12.

10

Pharmacologic Treatment

There is no cure for dystonia. Those cases that are secondary to medications, even tardive dystonia, may improve with time after discontinuation of the causative agent. For most primary dystonias, however, there are only treatments to alleviate the symptoms. However, this improvement is significant in most cases. Every patient and every case of dystonia is different, and thus the treatment plan appropriate for your case needs to be developed through cooperation with your treating physician.

This chapter discusses mainly oral medications, those taken by mouth. The common oral medications used for dystonias can be divided into pharmaceutical classes, each of which shares common mechanisms of action and, for the most part, a common group of side effects. These general characteristics are discussed for each class, and are accompanied by a listing of several commonly used medications within each. It is important to note that not all dystonias are treated the same; some of the medications described here are used only for certain types of dystonias.

ANTICHOLINERGICS

Acetylcholine is a chemical transmitter that is involved in controlling a number of involuntary functions in the body, including digestion, urination, and salivation. Drugs that increase levels of acetylcholine cause drooling, watery eyes, stomach cramps, diarrhea, the need to urinate, and sweating. Medications that interfere with the effects of acetylcholine, called anticholinergics, have the opposite effects, including dry mouth, constipation, difficulty urinating, drowsiness, and, at high doses, mental confusion. Fortunately, if doses of medications are started at low levels and then increased gradually, your body can get used to the side effects and they will diminish and become easier to tolerate.

Two commonly used anticholinergic medications are Artane (trihexphenidyl) and Cogentin (benztropine mesylate). At high doses, these medications provide mild-to-moderate relief of the muscle spasms and twisting, although they are not very effective at relieving pain. If you are currently using one of these medications and are not experiencing severe side effects, there are a few precautions you should take. You should stay out of extreme heat, as these medications reduce the ability to sweat, and you should drink plenty of fluids to counteract dry mouth and constipation. If you are having difficulty urinating while on these medications, consult your doctor.

SEDATIVES

Most sedative medications used for the treatment of dystonias are in a drug class known as benzodiazepines. The benzodiazepines most commonly used are Valium (diazepam), Ativan (lorazepam), Klonopin (clonazepam), and sometimes Xanax (alprazolam). Benzodiazepines are most commonly used in low doses as anxiety relieving medications. They are also sometimes used as prescription sleeping aids. At higher doses, they may be used to treat epileptic seizures or to calm severely agitated or violent patients. It is not known exactly how benzodiazepines improve dystonia, but they do have a muscle relaxing effect.

Sedation is the major side effect of benzodiazepines. Drowsiness in the evening is usually not a problem, but daytime drowsiness can be bothersome. One major concern patients have about being prescribed benzodiazepines is their potential to cause drug addiction. They may have heard of the names of some commonly used benzodiazepines as drugs that are used by drug abusers. When it occurs, addiction usually happens to patients taking the drugs for other diagnoses, such as anxiety disorder or behavior control. Addiction is very uncommon among dystonia patients. In fact, we have yet to see true addiction and abuse of benzodiazepines in any of our dystonia patients. An important distinction must be made here. *Addiction* is not the same as *dependence*. If a medication does what it is supposed to do and significantly reduces dystonia symptoms, then a patient may depend on it to function normally. Additionally, once the patient's motor system and brain have adapted to a certain dose of benzodiazepines, the medication should not be stopped abruptly. Abrupt discontinuation of medication may result in temporary worsening of symptoms (*rebound effect*), and other withdrawal symptoms such as seizures may occur.

ANTISPASTICITY MEDICATIONS

These medications are most often used to treat muscle spasticity that occurs in disorders of the primary, or *pyramidal*, motor system, such as strokes and spinal cord injuries. There are differences in the type of increased muscle tone seen in pyramidal motor system disorders versus extrapyramidal movement disorders, but these differences need not concern us at this point. These different divisions of the motor system are discussed in Chapter 2.

The first antispasticity medicine is baclofen. This medication is especially useful in patients with spastic limbs and brisk tendon-jerk reflexes. Its sedating side effects are more tolerable than those of benzodiazepines. Baclofen can be taken orally or can be delivered directly into the fluid surrounding the spinal cord and brain by means of a catheter that is attached to an electronically programmable pump, as discussed in the chapter on generalized dystonia.

Two other antispasticity medications belong to a family of drugs called *alpha receptor agonists*. The details of alpha receptor functions need not be discussed here. The exact way in which these reduce muscle spasms is not well defined. The two most common of these medications are Catapress (clonidine) and Zanaflex (tizanidine). Catapress is used most often as a blood pressure-lowering agent. Zanaflex is used for muscle spasticity, and to relieve muscle pain of the type associated with tension cervicalgia. Both are used for pyramidal spasticity and may be applied to extrapyramidal dystonias. The major side effects are sedation and low blood pressure, which may cause light-headedness when standing up. Zanaflex tends to relieve some pain associated with dystonias.

Another antispasticity medicine is Dantrium (dantrolene). This medication works within the cells of muscle tissue, inhibiting the contraction of those cells and thereby the contraction of the entire muscle. Doses of Dantrium high enough to diminish muscle spasms usually cause diffuse weakness in all the muscles of the body and usually produce sedation as well. For these reasons it is rarely employed for the treatment of focal dystonias, and our own experiences in prescribing it have not yielded very impressive results.

DOPAMINE-ENHANCING MEDICATIONS

Dopamine-enhancing medications work in a number of ways to increase the activity of dopamine in the extrapyramidal motor system. They are most often used to treat Parkinson disease, in which dopamine-producing neurons of the extrapyramidal system stop functioning and eventually die. Sinemet is a commonly used Parkinson disease medication that delivers a chemical called *levodopa* to the brain. Levodopa is subsequently converted to dopamine. Other medications, called *dopamine agonists*, deliver to the brain chemicals that behave very much like dopamine and have similar effects. Dopamine agonists include Mirapex (pramipexole), Requip (ropinirole), and Parlodel (bromocriptine). All of these medications are useful in treating patients who have DYT-5, or dopamine-responsive dystonia, described in Chapter 3. Side effects include nausea, loss of appetite, sedation, and constipation. Dopamine-enhancing medications should be tried for a brief period of time in appropriately selected dystonia patients. Unfortunately, only a tiny fraction of patients have a dopamine-responsive dystonia.

ANTIDEPRESSANTS

Medications in this class have a variety of different mechanisms of action. They are, of course, used to treat depression. If a dystonia patient also has associated depression, his or her doctor may choose to employ a medication from this class. Many of these medications have anticholinergic side effects, providing some relief from dystonia as well, though this benefit is smaller than that achieved with true anticholinergics. Apart from these effects, however, antidepressant medications have the property of reducing the symptoms of chronic pain, which is a frequent sequela of dystonia. The mechanism by which these medications relieve chronic pain is not known. However, because of this property they are sometimes used to alleviate chronic headaches as well as the pain from pinched nerves or other disorders of the peripheral nerves.

Side effects of antidepressants vary with the type used. The most frequently experienced side effect is sedation. Anticholinergic side effects such as dry mouth, constipation, and urinary retention are also experienced. The most commonly used antidepressants for pain belong to a family known as *tricyclic* antidepressants. These include Elavil (amitriptyline), Tofranil (imipramine), and Pamelor (nortriptyline). Tricyclic antidepressants may be the most effective for pain control, but they have greater side effects. Other antidepressants, called *selective serotonin reuptake inhibitors* (SSRIs), have fewer side effects, and their pain-relieving properties are still being elucidated. These include Zoloft (sertralene) and Paxil (paroxetine). Still other antidepressants, called *selective norepinephrine and serotonin reuptake inhibitors* (SNRIs), appear to have even better pain-relieving properties. These include Effexor (venlafaxine), Wellbutrin (bupropion), and Cymbalta (duloxetine).

THE STRATEGY OF ORAL MEDICATION THERAPY

As you have no doubt gleaned from reading the preceding sections, all of the medications used for dystonia seem to have limited benefit. Although a few people have an excellent response to one or more medications with great improvement of symptoms, the vast majority experiences only a mild or moderate relief of neck twisting and pain. Additionally, as you have no doubt noticed, most of the medications have significant side effects. If your doctor decides to try oral medications to treat your condition, he will choose a medication from the class best suited for you in terms of the severity of your condition and the presence of any other conditions that may require treatment. For example, in the presence of depression or significant nerve pain, an antidepressant medication may be the best choice for a first try. A brief trial of dopamine-enhancing medication may be appropriate for certain patients to avoid missing a case of dopamine-responsive dystonia. Anticholinergics and benzodiazepines are the most frequently chosen medications to treat dystonia.

Regardless of which medication is chosen, the motto for dosing is "start low and go slow." This means that the starting dose should be low enough to avoid intolerable side effects. The dose is usually increased slowly over a number of weeks, while the doctor and the patient monitor the occurrence and severity of side effects. Increasing the dose gradually allows the body to become used to the drug and to compensate for side effects. For example, the anticholinergic effect of dry mouth tends to diminish with time. The sedating side effects of many medications also diminish, allowing higher doses to be used.

The biggest reason many patients "fail" a medication trial is that they do not see any improvement in symptoms after the first few weeks. During this time, they may experience some side effects and then stop taking the drug. The initial low dose may not be enough to improve symptoms, but may cause some side effects. In general, it may take several weeks or even a few months of therapy to find out if a particular drug is going to be of any benefit. Our biggest concern in oral medication therapy is that a particular drug has been declared ineffective when, in fact, an adequate trial of appropriate duration and dose has not been done. If the first medication tried is not effective or is not tolerated, a second choice must be made and the process started again. Remember, dystonia is a chronic, usually life-long condition. It takes a great deal of patience and perseverance on the part of you and your doctor to find the most beneficial medication and dose.

PAIN CONTROL

Pain has been discussed as an integral component of dystonia, and we considered it as one of the "hidden symptoms" of dystonia. Medications used to treat the spasming muscles, usually Artane, Valium, or other benzodiazepines, also alleviate pain. However, supplementary treatments often are needed specifically for the pain. Pain in dystonia, especially cervical dystonia, responds well to treatment with botulinum toxin, discussed in Chapter 11.

First-line pain medications include anti-inflammatory analgesics, either in nonprescription or prescription strength. We generally choose ibuprofen (Advil, Motrin, others), or naproxen sodium (Aleve, Naprox, others). These medications are also our first choices for relieving any local injection site pain that may occur after botulinum toxin injections. As adjuncts to these, we may add medications that contain a narcotic analgesic substance, such as Vicodin, which contains hydrocodone. The list of medications that contain hydrocodone or a similar narcotic is long. We try to not prescribe narcotic pain medications on an "as needed" basis because the risks of both narcotic dependence and addiction are fairly high. We have noted that our dystonia patients who receive such medications have difficulty in discontinuing them.

For patients with persistent focal pain in one or two particular areas, injection of a local anesthetic agent, such as those used by dentists, to those tender, or "trigger," points can alleviate pain on a temporary basis. Lidocaine and bupivicaine are the most commonly used local anesthetic agents. Such local anesthetic injections, also referred to as "trigger point" injections, may be effectively used to keep pain at a tolerable level between scheduled botulinum toxin treatments, which are usually about three months apart. Finally, intrathecal pump implantation may be done to deliver pain medication, usually morphine or one of its derivatives, into the spinal fluid.

11

Chemodenervation/Botulinum Toxin

As you have learned, oral medications have limited benefit in dystonia patients and are difficult to use because of side effects. Fortunately, there is another way to reduce the over-contraction of muscles that are pulling and contorting the body. Surgery can be employed to cut nerves or muscles involved in dystonia, especially in cervical dystonia. The injection of a muscle-weakening agent into the spasming dystonic muscles can also block signals from motor nerves. This procedure is known as *chemodenervation.*

The injection of a muscle-weakening agent into the dystonic muscles can normalize abnormal posture, relieve spasms, and reduce pain. Chemodenervation agents work by disrupting motor nerve endings within a muscle. The muscle then cannot receive the signal to contract. The treated muscle becomes loose, slackened, or paralyzed for a prolonged period of time. Formerly, solvent chemicals such as *phenol* were used for chemodenervation. Although phenol still has useful applications, the agent most frequently used now is *botulinum toxin.* During the 1970s, this toxin was purified from bacteria cultures grown in a laboratory and then carefully processed for injection into muscle tissue for therapeutic medical use. The bacteria used are called *Clostridium botulinum.*

Present in an inactive form in our environment, *C. botulinum* thrives in airless, or *anaerobic,* conditions, such as inside poorly preserved or canned food, or in the depths of a dirty puncture wound. When it flourishes and becomes active under such conditions, it releases toxin that is poisonous to motor nerve endings. Persons who suffer this poisoning develop the disease called *botulism,* in which they become progressively weaker: their muscles become gradually flaccid and paralyzed and ultimately they can no longer move. When the breathing muscles collapse, death will ensue unless artificial mechanical respiration is begun. When placed on a respirator, the patient can be sustained until motor nerve endings regenerate, a process that may take months.

Botulinum toxin certainly sounds like a frightening substance to employ for medical therapy. Indeed, a poison possibly employed by the maharajas of ancient India—a tasteless powder extracted from dried meat—is likely to have contained botulinum toxin. As an assassination tool, it would have had the added benefit of a few days' delay before symptoms were noted, thus allaying suspicions from the poisoner. The U.S. military even researched its potential as a biological weapon of mass destruction during World War II. However, purified and carefully processed botulinum toxin has been used as a medical therapeutic agent since the early 1970s.

Purified botulinum toxin was first employed to treat a disorder of the eyes called *strabismus,* in which the two eyes are misaligned with one another. When injected into appropriate muscles behind the eyeball, it can correct this misalignment. It soon became apparent that botulinum toxin could be used to treat almost any medical condition that is characterized by increased muscle tone or abnormal muscle contraction in any part of the body. Dystonias and dyskinesias are primary among such disorders.

There are several strains, or subspecies, of *C. botulinum,* each of which produces its own variation of botulinum toxin. The different types of botulinum toxin are classified according to their chemical structure. Toxin type A is marketed in the United States under the brand name Botox. Recently Dysport, another botulinum toxin A, was approved by the FDA, although it has been used for over 20 years in other countries. Botulinum toxin type B is marketed in the United States under the name Myobloc. Other brands are available outside the United States and from different companies. These are all toxin type A, and include Xeomin, produced by Merz in Germany; Prosigne by Hengli, China; and Neuronox by Medy-Tox, South Korea. As of this writing, Xeomin is only available in the United States under research protocols. Prosigne and Neuronox are not available in the United States.

The first step in chemodenervation treatment is to determine which muscles need to be targeted for injection. From the knowledge of the anatomy and normal movement actions of various muscles, the physician can reasonably guess which muscles are involved. Your doctor may then examine the muscles by *palpation,* touching and pressing them to confirm which are abnormally contracting. In some cases, this is all that is necessary to establish the target muscles. In other cases, the target muscles may not be so obvious, and diagnostic testing may be necessary. Diagnostic testing usually consists of *electromyography* (EMG), in which a needle electrode is inserted into a suspect muscle and the electrical output of its muscle cells is recorded.

The next step is to determine the dose of botulinum toxin to be given to each muscle and the overall dose to be used for a particular patient. There is no set dose for each muscle or for any patient, although there are some rule-of-thumb guidelines. Larger muscles require higher doses than smaller muscles, and strongly contracting muscles require higher doses than moderately contracting ones. Additionally, the overall dose is determined by the physical size and muscularity of the patient. A large, athletically-built man will certainly require much more toxin than a slim, petite female. If too little toxin is given, there will be little beneficial effect, and any reduction of the symptoms will be short-lived. If excessive toxin is given, muscles may become too weak, and the patient may have difficulty using the limb or keeping the head upright. For these reasons, our practice is to start off with a mid-range or conservative dose. Although this may not provide maximum benefit, it allows us to assess how the patient responds to the treatment and safeguards against possible side effects.

Another complication in deciding the correct dose is that the measured units are not the same among the three formulations of botulinum toxin. Fifty units of Myobloc is not equivalent to 50 units of Botox or Dysport. In the end, your doctor must choose your doses based upon the severity of your dystonia, the muscles involved, your physical size, and the particular formulation of botulinum toxin he chooses to use. Sometimes, nearby muscles that were not injected will take over the function of chemodenervated muscles, resulting in a change in the pattern of the dystonia. This will require reassessment and modification of the treatment approach. It may take several subsequent treatments with various doses and targeted muscles before an optimal response is achieved, one that is effective without causing excessive weakness or side effects.

Botulinum toxin may be injected into target muscles through a conventional hypodermic needle. In some cases, a doctor may choose to deliver the injection through an electrically insulated conductive hypodermic needle attached to an EMG machine. Simultaneous recording of EMG muscle activity allows the doctor to know when the needle tip is exactly within the body of the target muscle. It takes approximately three days before the effects of botulinum toxin injections are noticed, and three-to-four weeks for maximum effect to be seen. After this, the effects begin to slowly wear off, as nerve endings within the muscles regenerate. The beneficial effect lasts for about three months, after which the injections must be repeated.

Chemodenervation by botulinum toxin injection is currently the most effective method of relieving the abnormal muscle spasms of many types of dystonias. The effectiveness in any dystonia patient depends on the severity of his or her condition. Some patients expect that their symptoms will continue to improve progressively with each successive treatment until the condition is completely resolved. This is unfortunately not the case. Symptoms return as the effect of botulinum toxin wears off. For instance, suppose a patient with a rotational torticollis of 60 degrees receives chemodenervation treatment and that the rotation subsequently improves to 30 degrees. As the toxin's effect wears off over time, the patient's head will slowly drift back approximately to the original 60 degrees of rotation. Subsequent chemodenervation treatments should have about the same effect as the first one, improving the rotation to approximately 30 degrees. Subsequent treatments will not progressively improve rotation until neutral position (zero degrees) is reached. A few patients have even noticed that the results from their first chemodenervation were the best, and that subsequent treatments did not produce the same degree of improvement. This phenomenon has many explanations, which may vary from individual to individual.

Sometimes, a patient who has had a stable level of improvement with each botulinum toxin injection will notice a loss of effectiveness after several years of treatment. This may be due to the development of antibodies that make an individual resistant to the botulinum toxin. The more frequently injections are given and the higher the toxin dose at each treatment, the greater is the tendency for an individual to develop resistance antibodies. Therefore, it is recommended that injections be given no more frequently than every three months and that the lowest effective dose be used at each treatment. It is noteworthy that the incidence of development of antibodies to botulinum toxin have markedly diminished since the introduction of the new purified botulinum toxin type A. Patients who develop resistance to one type of toxin may subsequently respond to injection of a different type. For example, Myobloc may be effective after Botox has stopped being effective.

Minor side effects from botulinum toxin injections include local redness and slight bruising from the injection needle. Some patients experience temporary numbness in the treated area. Remote side effects include dry mouth or dry eyes. Patients may experience "flu-like" symptoms of fatigue, muscle ache, body ache, or headache after injections. As with any injected medication, a local skin infection or allergic medication reaction is possible. However, sterile needles and alcohol wipes have nearly eliminated the occurrence of infection. Allergic reactions to botulinum toxin are very rare with the purified formulations currently used.

By far the most common side effects of botulinum toxin relate to overweakening of the target muscles or unintentional weakening of adjacent muscles as the toxin spreads through tissues surrounding the injection site. In the case of eye injections, such toxin diffusion can cause eyelid droop or double vision. In the case of neck muscle injection, it can cause droopiness of the head, with increasing neck pain as the patient strains the weakened muscles to keep his head upright. Another side effect of neck muscle injection is swallowing difficulty if the toxin diffuses to muscles of the voice box and throat. Overweakening of limb muscles can result in difficulty using that body part for necessary tasks. In all cases, problems caused by excessive muscle weakening resolve over two or three weeks, as the effects of the toxin begin to wear off. This type of side effect is avoidable at the next round of injections if the doctor reduces the dose or modifies the selection of target muscles.

12

Deep Brain Stimulation

■

My journey with dystonia began in mid-1988. I was a 23-year-old woman soon to be married, and was anticipating the start of my new life.

I began noticing some pulling sensations coming from the muscles in my trunk and shoulders. I would walk up to a mirror and see that I was slightly hunched over. This progressed, and I started walking around with my hands in the pockets of my pants to try to keep myself upright. I soon became pregnant with my first child in early 1989. I still had no clue what was happening to my body, and I finally took a permanent medical leave from my job in mid-1989. At this point, I was walking with a cane to help me get around. At home, I was actually bent over supporting myself with my hand on my knee to walk. And this was with a pregnant belly! I had a beautiful, healthy baby girl in December.

Many doctor visits marked my path to finding a diagnosis. But, you see, I was in a certain denial because I think I knew it was dystonia all along. Why? Because, my younger brother had been diagnosed with dystonia as a teenager. Our symptoms at that point were somewhat different, though.

In 1990 I met my brother's physician, who diagnosed me with generalized dystonia. It was hard to accept such a cruel intrusion of my body, but I knew I had to be optimistic and trust him. Years passed by with trial and error with many medications and lots of botulinum toxin injections. In 1994, I again became pregnant and had a very different and more enjoyable pregnancy, delivering another healthy, beautiful baby girl.

I seemed to have a euphoric period with botulinum toxin. Then, in 2000, I developed immunity to both botulinum toxin type A and later also to type B. I started on a slow downhill spiral again. My gait and walking were terrible and I had so, so many spasms.

The option of DBS was presented to me in the summer of 2004. I was somewhat leery of it and excited at the same time. By the end of August 2004 I had completed the entire process of DBS and within 2 months of adjustments I was walking erect and maintaining a normal gait. I was thrilled!

Since DBS, I have returned to life as I knew it when I was 21 years old. I consider my DBS experience a success story, but know and accept that dystonia is still a part of my life. The major thing that has changed is that dystonia is NOT my life now.

MEDICAL PERSPECTIVE

Deep brain stimulation (DBS) is a form of treatment for several medically refractory movement disorders including Parkinson disease, essential tremor, and dystonia. It is a form of brain surgery during which an electrode is placed into a part of the brain. The electrode is connected to a wire that runs under the skin of the scalp and neck and is attached to a battery-operated pulse generator the size of a small bar of hand soap that is implanted under the skin of the chest just below the collarbone. Electrical current from the pulse generator then stimulates the targeted site in the brain. It is not known exactly how the current dampens tremor and dystonia, but it is thought to inhibit, either directly or by inducing chemical changes, the brain activity that causes the involuntary movement. When the electrode is positioned in the appropriate brain site in the appropriate patient, DBS is a very effective form of treatment.

The target site for DBS electrode placement in dystonia can be either the thalamus or the globus pallidus. The thalamus acts as a relay station for the brain messages to and from the body. DBS in the thalamus improves tremor and sometimes also helps with writer's cramp, a form of focal dystonia. There are limitations to using this site. It is usually performed only on one side (the side opposite the tremor) so as not to cause problems with gait, speech, and memory. More severe forms of dystonia respond to DBS in the globus pallidus.

The globus pallidus is the part of the basal ganglia in the brain where it appears dystonia originates. Placing electrodes in the globus pallidus on both sides of the brain can be helpful to treat generalized and segmental dystonia. The best response tends to occur in patients with hereditary forms of dystonia. Severe cervical dystonia that does not respond to botulinum toxin injections may respond to DBS. But DBS does not help everyone with dystonia. We are not advanced enough in our knowledge of dystonia and this treatment to be able to help in every case. Sometimes people with dystonia do not derive any benefit despite going through the brain surgery and the best attempts at adjusting the stimulator. And brain surgery is just that: brain surgery. There are risks with any surgery and brain surgery is not without exception. There is a risk of bleeding in the brain and stroke. In addition, speech and walking can also be affected even in the absence of other surgical complications.

DBS surgery usually takes place in stages, sometimes separated by a week. In the first stage, a circular metal frame called a *halo* is screwed into the skull and an MRI is obtained of the head with attached frame. Then, with the assistance of a computer, the surgeon plots the location of targets in the image of the brain in relation to reference points on the halo. Holes are drilled into the skull and, using the metal halo as a guide, the surgeon places the electrode at the correct angle and depth to reach the previously plotted target. The patient is awake during this part and will be asked to cooperate during testing of the electrode. For example they will be asked to speak, move their hand, and so on. This is important because the neurosurgeon wants to be certain the electrode is in the right place before finishing this stage of the surgery. After this, the halo is removed.

The second stage involves connecting the electrode's attached wire from the outside of the skull to the pulse generator and battery. The wires are tunneled under the skin and attached to the pulse generator, which is implanted under the skin of the chest below the collarbone.

PATIENT PERSPECTIVE

Just before undergoing that surgery, we went for a last appointment to finalize preparations. As Kris and I were sitting in the reception room waiting to be seen, a man came out of one of the examination rooms. He could barely walk; his poor body was curled from the effects of dystonia. I looked at my daughter and said, "You know, even though you have the problems you do, it can always be worse." She looked at me and agreed.

DBS has opened a whole new world for Kris. When she first received the benefits of DBS she was like a little girl. She could write normally for the first time in years. She would sign her name over and over trying to decide which way she liked best. She could shave her legs pain free, no nicks and cuts. She could eat with chopsticks. There are a million little things she can do now that we all take for granted. So at 34 years of age, Kris is starting a new phase in her life.

There are a few inconveniences she has to endure. The battery for the DBS system doesn't last very long. She has to undergo outpatient surgery every 13 to 15 months to replace the unit. She has to be sure to catch the timing right because if the battery dies before it's replaced, her symptoms come back tenfold. For air travel, she has to go through a separate security line because she can't walk through the regular electronic system. There is a bulge under her skin on the right side of her chest. It looks exactly like a cell phone stuck just below the skin. At first she was very self-conscious about the scar and the bulge, but now she just accepts it being there. To me, it's like a badge of honor. It stands for all the trials and tribulations she has gone through and will go through until they find some other means to handle her dystonia. It has been now 6 years that she got her life back. For us this is like a second life.

After surgery, the device needs to be programmed. For dystonia, the electrical output settings are high and require long periods of time before improvement starts. On average it takes about 3 months before improvement of the dystonia begins. Symptoms continue to improve gradually over time. Sometimes the improvement allows discontinuation of any medications the patient is taking for the dystonia. The response can be dramatic and patients can return to their previous levels of activity. However, the high output settings required shorten the battery life span, which is usually less than 2 years. That means the battery will need to be replaced every 2 years. A new form of battery has just become available that may improve this situation. This is a rechargeable battery that lasts 9 years. However, the patient needs to wear a device to recharge the battery every day for 15 minutes. The battery cannot be allowed to run out of energy or it will have to be replaced. If you are considering this treatment for your form of dystonia, please consult your movement disorders specialist or neurologist.

13

Cervical Dystonia or Spasmodic Torticollis

PATIENT PERSPECTIVE

Sam first began to notice head shaking when he was 40 years of age. In fact, his family first noticed he was shaking his head as if in disagreement several months before he realized something was wrong. They noticed that his head shook off and on, especially when he was driving. His coworkers also noticed this and wondered why he shook his head "no" so often even when he was saying "yes" verbally. Sam did not realize his head was shaking until one day he noticed he was looking to the right all the time. It became more difficult to watch television unless his head was supported on the back of his favorite recliner. He wasn't able to read the paper at the breakfast table and had to retreat back to his recliner to do so. He began to have difficulty driving and tended to rest his head on the headrest in order to look straight ahead. He went to his family doctor, who told Sam that he did not know what was wrong and prescribed a course of physical therapy.

Sam completed the physical therapy despite feeling worse after the more rigorous exercise, and was no better. Although the head turning was uncomfortable and caused him problems, he decided that there wasn't anything else to do for this condition and resolved to continue the exercises and live with it. Gradually, his neck returned to the neutral position and he remained symptom free for the next 20 years. Then, while he was walking for exercise, Sam noticed his head again pulling to the right. This time, his family doctor sent him to a neurologist specializing in movement disorders, who diagnosed Sam as having cervical dystonia.

MEDICAL PERSPECTIVE

A number of different medical conditions may cause an abnormal head and neck posture, and the term *cervical dystonia* or *torticollis* has loosely been applied to many of them. In fact, torticollis simply means "twisted neck." This chapter deals specifically with the neurological movement disorder known as *cervical dystonia* (CD), also known as *spasmodic torticollis* (ST). Other causes of abnormal neck posture will be briefly discussed to differentiate them from CD. The term cervical dystonia is technically more correct, although spasmodic torticollis is commonly used. The neck is also known by its Latin name, *cervix*, and from there the term *cervical dystonia* derives. For purposes of the discussion in this chapter, we provide the following definition: CD is a *neurological* disorder that results in an involuntary turning or twisting of the head and neck, forcing the patients to assume an abnormal posture. It is difficult for the person with CD to voluntarily move his or her head back to a normal straight position. The word *involuntary* should be stressed here. This means that the affected individual is not voluntarily, or volitionally, moving his or her head into the abnormal posture. He or she may have to exert voluntary effort to try to bring the head back to normal position, but when that effort is stopped, his or her head will return to the abnormal position.

Now that you have an understanding of the definition of CD, we will go over the signs and symptoms of this disorder in more detail. CD may begin at any age, but appears most often between the ages 25 and 55 years. It affects men and women about equally, and has no predilection for any particular race or ethnic group. The disorder usually develops gradually. Neck discomfort, mild pain, and a feeling of stiffness may be the earliest symptoms. Muscle contractions may produce subtle jerking movements of the head that resemble a tremor. These early manifestations may not be present all of the time. They may occur only when the individual is fatigued, such as at the end of the day, or may appear transiently during or after physical stress or exercise, or during anxiety or emotional stress. There may be a subtle tilt to the head, but individuals at this stage are seldom aware of their torticollis as a distinct medical disorder. They usually believe they are experiencing "muscle tension," and treat themselves with over-the-counter pain medications, massage, rest, and sometimes chiropractic care.

When the symptoms persist, sufferers may see their primary physician. Unless the signs of the disorder are obvious at this point, they may then, appropriately, receive conservative treatments with prescription pain medications, muscle relaxants, and possibly refer-ral to a physical therapist or chiropractor. Sometimes, in mild cases, these conservative measures may be all that are required to keep the symptoms at a reasonably tolerable level, even if a definitive diagnosis of ST has not been made. In many cases, however, the disorder progresses over months, or even a few years. The symptoms become more continuous and persistent. Head and neck position becomes more contorted and the abnormal posture is obvious to the patient and to others. Pain and stiffness may increase, and pain medications or muscle relaxants may no longer be effective. It becomes increasingly difficult to voluntarily move the head back to neutral position. Head tremor may increase, resembling a nodding "yes-yes" or a shaking "no-no" motion. Occasionally, the dystonia can spread to adjacent body parts such as the shoulders, arms, hands, or the back and spine.

Depending on the severity that the disorder eventually reaches, the twisted posture and pain begin to interfere with a person's normal functioning. An affected person might have trouble shaving, combing his or her hair, or applying makeup. It may become more difficult to read, watch television, or drive. Job performance may be impaired. Social interactions may also suffer. This may be due to the individual's own self-conscious embarrassment. It can also be due to aversion or avoidance by strangers, coworkers, or acquaintances; the individual may be assumed by others to have a psychiatric disorder.

Occasionally, especially early in the course of the disease, symptoms of CD will spontaneously remit. In a few cases, remission may be complete and permanent. In the majority of cases, however, the symptoms will reappear at a later date, and the CD becomes a chronic permanent disorder. The general observation has been made that the greater the length of time that symptoms have been present, the more likely that the condition will be permanent. The CD almost never resolves if symptoms have been present for more than one or two years. Its slow progression usually reaches a plateau after about five years, at which point symptoms become stable.

In the chronic stage, the severity of symptoms varies from day to day. Symptoms tend to worsen with fatigue, heavy exercise, and stress, while sleep and relaxation tend to reduce them. Many people find relief by lying on their back, although this is not true for everyone. The neck movements always stop during sleep and for some people do not reappear for a period of time after awakening. The term "honeymoon period" was coined by Dr. Daniel Truong in the 1980s to describe this period after awakening, during which the patient's CD is not present. It can last from a few minutes to a few hours. The length of the honeymoon period tends to shrink as time goes by. Neck pain may become the predominant symptom.

PAIN

Pain is one of the "hidden symptoms" in CD patients. While abnormal head posture or tremor is obvious to other people, pain is not. The incessant continuous muscle contractions in CD result in severe fatigue, producing pain in the involved muscles. This pain resembles what many of us have experienced during a "charley horse" cramp in the leg or foot. It can also resemble the muscle soreness that occurs after we perform exercise to which we are not accustomed. Such pain and soreness are temporary conditions for most people, but they are continuous in people with CD. Pain is generated by a number of mechanisms. The bones, joints, ligaments, muscles, and other tissues of your neck all have sensory nerve endings that send input signals, including pain impulses, centrally to the spinal cord and sensory portions of your brain. Chronic spasmodic contraction of a muscle stimulates the sensory nerve endings within it. Chronic torsion of joints, ligaments, and other tissues creates shearing and stretching forces in some places, and squeezing or compression in others. This also stimulates nerve endings in those areas.

Additionally, the chronic torsional forces can hasten the development of arthritic changes in the joints between vertebral bones. Some arthritic changes involve overgrowth of bone at the edges of joints, which may then impinge on nerves entering or exiting the cervical spine. The rubbery disks interposed between each of the cervical vertebrae can also become affected. Abnormalities of these discs are more common in CD sufferers than in otherwise healthy people. The discs can become compressed or flattened. At the same time, the edges of the discs can bulge outward into the central spinal canal.

If the bulging is severe, it can compress the motor and sensory nerves attached to the spinal cord, especially if there is also bony arthritic overgrowth in the area. Spinal nerve root compression is called *radiculopathy*, and it is likely to cause *radicular pain* that radiates outward toward the shoulder or arm. If motor nerves become severely compressed, those shoulder and arm muscles that they supply may become weak or shrunken (atrophied), leading to loss of ability to use the arm. Extreme disc bulging can even narrow the central canal and impinge on the spinal cord.

All of these factors combine to create pain. The severity of pain experienced by CD patients varies widely and does not always correspond to the severity of the abnormal position. Pain also tends to worsen with fatigue or after physical exertion. For many people with CD, pain is just as disabling, if not more disabling, as the abnormal head posture or tremor. Fortunately, severe radicular pain, muscle atrophy, and spinal cord impingement only occur in severe cases. Chronic pain is a serious condition. It can hamper your concentration at work and at other tasks. It can destroy your motivation to perform all of those activities needed to live and enjoy your life. Chronic pain can create a state of apathy and even lead to clinical depression.

Fortunately, treatments that alleviate spasmodic muscle contraction and improve head position also alleviate pain. Pain responds well to chemodenervation by injection of botulinum toxin. In addition, other methods both conventional and nonconventional may be used to manage pain; these are discussed in Chapter 10.

GESTE ANTAGONISTE: THE "SENSORY TRICK"

Many people with CD develop a tendency to place their hand on the side of their neck or place their fingers against their chin or cheek. For some reason, a light sensory stimulus on the skin of the head or neck dampens the tremors and reduces the severity of the twisting, making it easier to volitionally hold the head in a neutral position. This is known as a "sensory trick," or *geste antagoniste*. Most patients discover this for themselves without needing to be taught. They tend to use this method when reading, watching television, or eating. Unfortunately, the effect of the geste antagoniste is temporary, and full symptoms return as soon as the stimulus is removed. The sensory trick has different levels of effect for different individuals, and not everyone can benefit from it. The exact location of the area to be used and the way in which it is pressed or touched also differs. Some people find relief by putting a hand on the back of their neck. This may also be considered a geste antagoniste, although its mechanism of benefit may be different, having more to do with supporting the head. Some people may also find relief by lying down on their back. If you have not yet found an effective sensory trick, it may take some experimentation to find one that is effective for you.

■

PATIENT PERSPECTIVE

Through my experience, I've noted the importance of a proper diagnosis by a qualified neurologist with a specialty in movement disorders. For the most part, internists, family/general physicians, and orthopedic surgeons do not recognize the disease, and it often goes on for years being either undiagnosed or misdiagnosed. I was very fortunate because I worked in the medical field and was able to be diagnosed right away by a neurologist who recognized the disorder. The first step in the right direction of being able to cope with CD is proper diagnosis. I was referred to a university facility and enrolled in a research program for botulinum toxin, which at the time I was diagnosed, botulinum toxin was still in its research phase and not yet approved by the FDA.

PHYSIOLOGY

Before we get into details about the causes and mechanics of CD, we'll need some basic lessons on how muscles and joints work and how they are controlled by the nervous system.

It is believed that the human brain has a "set point" for the natural, neutral resting position of the head and neck, with the face pointing forward, the head and chin level, and the neck following a slight natural curve. The extrapyramidal system integrates all of the sensory input information discussed above to maintain just the right amount of balanced resting tone in the neck muscles to keep the head on an "even keel." In CD, the normal "set point" becomes altered in the brain. The mechanism how this occurs is not yet known.

ANATOMY AND MECHANICS OF THE NECK

The neck is one of the most remarkably agile and flexible parts of your body, partly because it must compensate for the visual limitation of having your eyes in the front of your head. Let us look at some of the mechanics of head and neck motion. Your skull rests on top of a column of neck bones, or *vertebrae*. Each vertebra is separated from the ones above and below it by a flexible rubberlike disk. The column of vertebrae and interposed disks is called the *cervical spine* (Figure 1). You can rotate your head left or right and bend it forward or sideways. Most of the rotation occurs between the first two cervical vertebrae from the top. Bending occurs to some degree between all of them. Several muscles connect your cervical spine with your skull, and the bones of your shoulder girdle with your cervical spine and skull.

The resting tone of these muscles maintains your head and neck position. When you want to *voluntarily* move your head in any particular direction, your brain chooses an appropriate set of these muscles to contract and pull your head into the desired new position. When the "set point" becomes altered in the brain, as in CD, some muscles become involuntarily overactive. The result is that instead of the normal balanced resting tone of neck muscles, overactive contractions of a set of muscles pull the head and neck into an abnormal or contorted posture that approximates the new "set point." For purposes of our discussion in the rest of this book, we

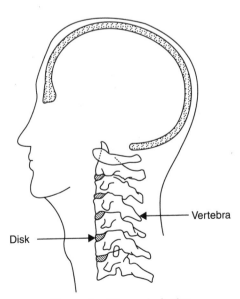

Figure 1 *The cervical spine.*

will refer to the primary set of overactive, involuntarily contracting muscles as *agonists*. Other neck muscles may be used, voluntarily or involuntarily, to attempt to correct head position back toward a normal resting posture. These muscles we will refer to as *antagonists*. Depending on the particular set of agonist muscles involved, the head and neck may assume a variety of abnormal postures. The normal movement of the neck is complex, and can include forward bending (*flexion*), backward bending (*extension*), right or left turning (*rotation*), and right or left tilting (*lateral*) movements. Thus, a case of CD can be described in terms of six major directional components: *anterocollis* (flexion, Figure 2), *retrocollis* (extension, Figure 3), right or left *torticollis* (rotation, Figure 4), and right or left *lateralcollis* (tilting, Figure 5). In addition to these major directional components, CD may also involve a shifting of the head forward or backward, or to either side. In the latter case, it may appear as though the shoulder toward which the head is shifted is shorter than the other. CD may be simple, involving only one direction, or it may be complex, involving more than one component—for example, a right rotation combined with a left tilt (Figure 6).

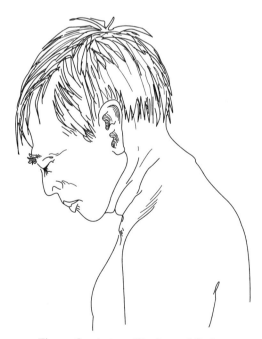

Figure 2 *Anterocollis, forward flexion.*

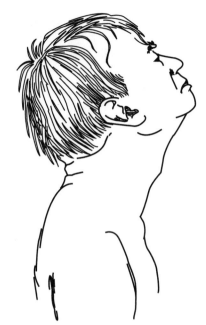

Figure 3   *Retrocollis, backwards extension.*

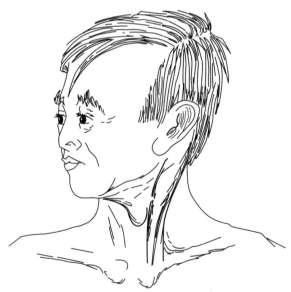

Figure 4   *Torticollis, rotation.*

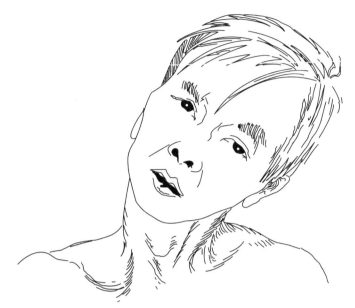

Figure 5 *Lateralcollis, tilting.*

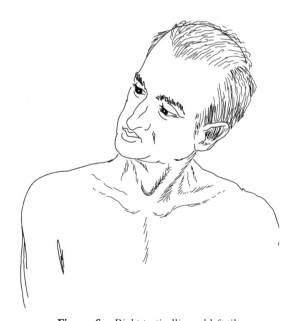

Figure 6 *Right torticollis and left tilt.*

THE MUSCLES INVOLVED IN CERVICAL DYSTONIA

One of the muscles most commonly involved in CD is the *sternocleido-mastoid* (SCM). This muscle stretches from the collarbone diagonally upwards along the front and side of your neck to insert on your skull just behind your ear (Figure 7). Contracting and shortening the length of your *right* SCM will rotate your face toward the *left*, while tucking your chin down toward your left collar bone (Figure 8). Contracting both of your SCM muscles will pull your head straight forward in flexion, tucking your chin into your chest. Other deeper muscles in the front of the neck are also involved in flexion.

The *trapezius* is a large, sheetlike triangular muscle that stretches from the cervical spine to the bones of the shoulder girdle (Figure 9). Contracting your right trapezius will pull the point of your right shoulder upwards and closer to your cervical spine, and also shift your head slightly to the right (Figure 10).

Another muscle that raises the point of your shoulder is the *levator scapuli* (Figure 11). This muscle starts on your cervical spine and runs downward to insert along the top of your shoulder blade. It can

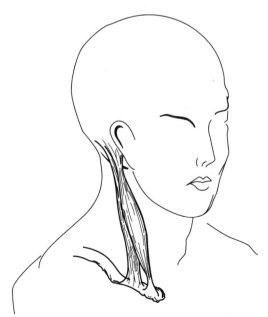

Figure 7 *The sternocleidomastoid muscle.*

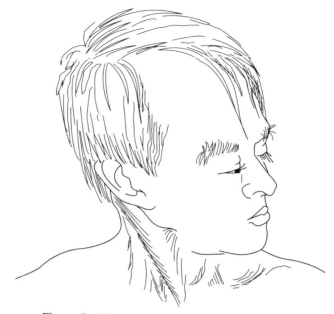

Figure 8   *The action of the right sternocleidomastoid.*

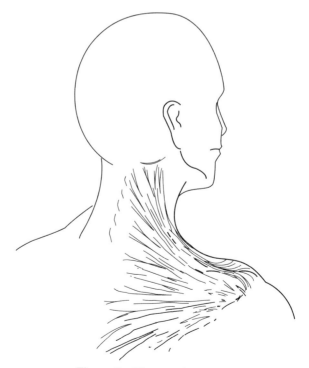

Figure 9   *The trapezius muscle.*

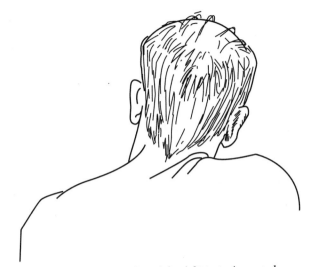

Figure 10 *The action of the right trapezius muscle.*

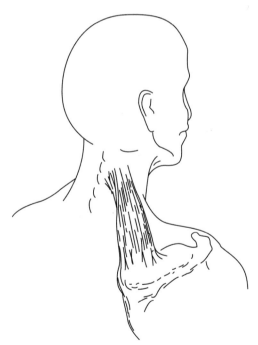

Figure 11 *The levator scapuli muscle.*

be felt at the base, or nape, of your neck just underneath the sheet of the trapezius. You can contract both of your trapezius and both of your levator scapuli muscles if you shrug both of your shoulders upwards as if to indicate "I don't know" with body language.

Another principal muscle is the *splenius capitis* (SC) in the back of your neck, which runs from the midline of the lower cervical spine diagonally upward to the base of your skull behind your ear (Figure 12). The pair of right and left SC muscles form a "V" in the back of the neck. The SC muscles lie in a layer underneath the broad sheet of the trapezius, which is more superficial (closer to the skin). Contracting your right SC will rotate your face toward the right, and partially tilt your head backwards in extension, moving your chin upward, away from your chest (Figure 13). Contracting both SC muscles will pull your head straight backwards in extension (Figure 14).

Other muscles, lying deeper to the SC, such as the semispinalis capitis and splenius cervicis, also contribute to neck extension.

The *scalenes* are a smaller set of muscles running vertically at the side of your neck, between the back edge of your SCM and the forward edge of your levator scapuli (Figure 15). The scalenes can be seen in some thin people, but are often difficult to find. Along with muscles

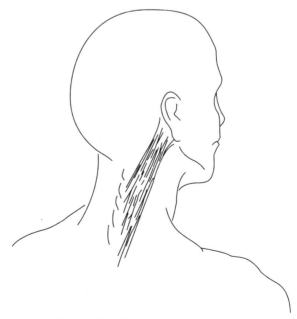

Figure 12 *The splenius capitis muscle.*

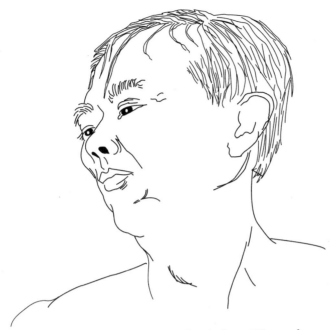

Figure 13   *The action of the right splenius capitis muscle.*

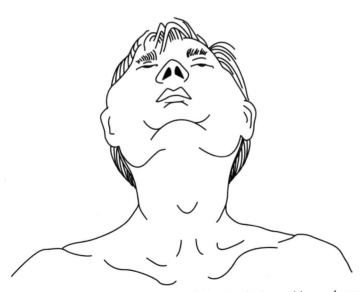

Figure 14   *Backward extension produced by both splenius capitis muscles and other posterior cervical muscles.*

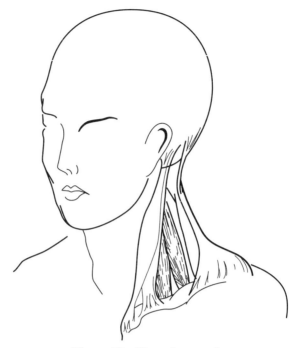

Figure 15 *The scalene muscles.*

such as the SCM and others, they tilt your head sideways, bringing your ear toward your shoulder (see Figure 5). The sets of muscles we have just discussed are the principal ones involved in most cases of ST. Many smaller or deeper muscles also play a part. As previously discussed, there are six primary directions in which your head moves: flexion, extension, right or left rotation, and right or left tilting. Most CD patients do not have just one abnormally contracting agonist muscle. They also do not commonly have a "pure" anterocollis, retrocollis, or torticollis. Usually, a set of several muscles is overactive, producing a complex head and neck posture; for example, a left torticollis with a right lateralcollis and a slight retrocollis, a posture resulting mainly from the actions of the right SCM and left SC (Figure 16).

THE CAUSES OF CERVICAL DYSTONIA

Primary Cervical Dysonia

It is not known why the extrapyramidal system goes awry and produces CD. The majority of cases of CD are primary, or idiopathic,

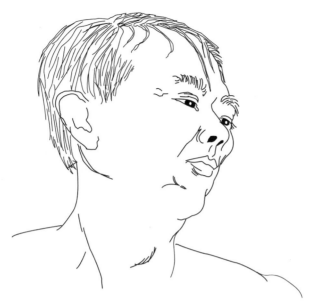

Figure 16 *The actions of right sternocleidomastoid and left splenius capitis muscles.*

meaning that they arise spontaneously in an individual with no identifiable cause or precipitating event. Idiopathic CD usually begins after 45 years of age. People with idiopathic CD are those most likely (about one in five) to have a spontaneous remission. The younger the age at onset of CD, the higher the chance is for spontaneous remission. Remissions usually last for a few years, even a decade in some cases. Unfortunately, the permanent disorder will ultimately reemerge in almost everyone with remission. The geste antagoniste works best for idiopathic CD patients. They tend also to have honeymoon periods. Placing the head or neck on a rest tends to relieve their symptoms. Their dystonia tends to remain limited to the head and neck muscles. Neck pain is mild or moderate in severity.

Inherited forms of dystonia usually begin in childhood and tend to involve the entire body. For instance, Oppenheim dystonia, discussed in Chapter 3, may manifest as CD in some family members. Other inherited cases of torticollis begin later in life, around 50 years of age, and tend to remain focal (localized to the head and neck).

PATIENT PERSPECTIVE

Grace first noticed some discomfort in her neck when she was 55 years of age. She was unable to maintain a neutral head position and would feel more comfortable with her head laid back while reading, watching television, or driving. She had difficulty reading, with her head pulling upwards while she read. Her head gradually began to pull to the right, with her chin rising, and she wasn't able to turn her head to the left easily. When her head became continually turned to the right, she developed pain in the neck and shoulder blade as well as headaches. She discovered her geste antagoniste; she found that placing her right hand on the right side of her face helped her to turn her head left. She later noted that her head turning was made worse after repetitive activity.

Recently she has developed a "shaky" quality to her voice, which worsens with prolonged talking or singing high notes. Her older sister experienced similar problems two years earlier. This led Grace to seek treatment for CD.

Several of Grace's family members suffer from dystonias. Two brothers and one older sister have been diagnosed with CD, and her mother and uncle had symptoms of head tremor and neck turning. Among her five children, her youngest son suffers from CD. Fortunately, Grace and her sister, who are both receiving treatment for CD, have had good responses and are now able to maintain a neutral head position.

Secondary Cervical Dystonia

In addition to idiopathic and genetic causes, there are a number of ways by which dystonia affecting the neck may be acquired, in which case it is considered *secondary* to another primary causative factor. Many of the diseases and external agents causing secondary dystonias have been described in Chapter 4. Tardive dyskinesia, caused by dopamine blocking medications, is one of the most common among these. After first reducing or eliminating the causative medications, tardive movement disorders may be treated by the same methods as primary CD; however, they do not respond as well to these treatments.

We must at this point also exclude those neck injury patients who have sustained orthopedic injury to the cervical spine, causing a dislocation or fracture of any of the vertebrae. This *orthopedic* condition will not be discussed here. However, physical trauma without spine fracture or dislocation can produce the *neurological* condition of cervical dystonia. In the early 1990s, Dr. Daniel Truong, one of the authors of this book, reported a small number of trauma-induced CD cases in the medical literature. These patients shared many similar characteristics, which are typified in the description of trauma-induced CD given below.

Since that first report, other cases were reported. Typically, individuals who develop trauma-induced CD have a mild-to-moderate neck trauma from falling, being struck in the neck, or suddenly catching or lifting a heavy object. Sometimes they have had a "whiplash" type injury. They sometimes report hearing a "snap" or "crack" at the time of the injury. Typically, they begin having neck pain and a feeling of stiffness immediately afterwards. Within weeks to a few months, they begin to develop abnormal neck posture, most often a lateral tilting toward one shoulder, and continued or increased pain. X-rays and other imaging studies do not reveal the fracture or dislocation of any neck bones.

In comparison to people with idiopathic CD, trauma-induced CD patients often don't experience any relief of symptoms with headrest or support. The geste antagoniste is not as effective in relieving their symptoms. Pain is a more severe component of their disorder. Medical treatments for CD do not work as well for these individuals as for those with the idiopathic disorder. In particular, treatment with botulinum toxin does not work as well. A greater percentage of them become limited in their activities or disabled and unable to work.

The importance of trauma as a causative factor in CD has been debated in the neurologic community for many years and remains a point of controversy. There are convincing arguments that some degree of sudden neck strain or minor trauma occurs frequently in the lives of active people, and that when one of them develops CD, there is a tendency to want to attribute it to an external cause. The issue is further complicated because many people who claim a traumatic cause are involved in litigation over the trauma and its resulting after-effects.

Neck trauma, whiplash, and similar injuries are common events. Certainly, only a tiny fraction of all such injuries results in the development of CD. It is not clear why very few people who sustain such a trauma develop CD while the vast majority do not. Some among this small number may have a genetic predisposition to develop movement disorders. It is also not clear how a relatively minor neck trauma can induce changes in the basal ganglia and extrapyramidal motor output of the brain to result in CD. It may be that the trauma disrupts the normal sensory inputs from muscles and joints of the neck to the brain and thus changes the information the brain uses to maintain its "set point" for head position. We can say that, among the hundreds of dystonia patients seen in our clinic over the years, we have identified only a handful who appear to have CD caused by trauma. In those cases that we have identified, CD symptoms began within days of the injury. Given that almost all of us have experienced a number of falls, tumbles, or neck strains at different times in our lives, there is no way to know whether an injury in the remote past has resulted in CD for any individual.

PATIENT PERSPECTIVE

Jake was 20 years of age when he was working in the tire industry. One day while lifting a large truck tire, he felt an abrupt pain in his neck. He immediately noticed that his neck was turned to the right, with his head tilted towards his right shoulder. He was unable to turn his head, and when he needed to look to the left, he had to turn his whole body in that direction. Because the pain in his neck was so severe, he went to a chiropractor and had physical therapy, which included massage and wearing some form of a harness that was designed to help straighten out his neck. He had no significant improvement with these treatments. He continued to work in a warehouse, however, managing as best as he could in an attempt to prevent total disability. Jake saw many doctors as well. He was once diagnosed as having Parkinson disease, but the medications prescribed for Parkinson disease did not work for him. This disorder had a major emotional impact on Jake's life. He had practically no social contact and only one date in 27 years. He started drinking alcohol in an attempt to help alleviate his pain and became an alcoholic. Twenty-seven years after the onset, Jake consulted a neurologist who specialized in CD and was subsequently treated with injections of botulinum toxin. His life was changed. This was the first time he experienced some pain relief. He stopped drinking alcohol, became more socially involved, and eventually married.

DIAGNOSIS OF CERVICAL DYSTONIA

CD is a rare disorder as medical illnesses go. It is estimated that only about three people out of 10,000 have some degree of CD. A primary care physician may thus only see one case of CD in several years, and that may be a mild case that is not easily recognized. Couple this with the fact that most patients walking into a doctor's office with a cocked head and neck pain are actually suffering from transient muscle strain or "wry neck," discussed below, or one of the orthopedic or other neurologic disorders that can mimic CD. Such a patient may, appropriately, receive treatment with analgesic pain medications, muscle relaxant medications, heat, ice, massage, physical therapy, or even chiropractic care. In many mild cases, these conservative measures alone may make the symptoms tolerable or acceptable, even if the definitive diagnosis of CD is not made.

If such conservative measures do not work, the patient may be referred to an orthopedic specialist. Those patients who have orthopedic causes can then receive the appropriate treatment. Certain patients suspected of having exposure to psychiatric medications may be referred to a psychiatrist. In fact, people with drug-induced dystonia of the neck are probably more common overall in the medical setting than true primary CD patients. This is probably the reason that CD is perceived as a psychiatric illness, or that CD patients are presumed to have an underlying psychiatric disorder. Whether a true CD patient is initially referred to an orthopedist or psychiatrist, he or she should eventually be suspected of having a neurologic disorder and be referred to a neurologist.

■

PATIENT PERSPECTIVE

Helen was 35 years of age when she began to notice pain in the left side of her neck and back of her head. She thought she was having headaches and treated herself with over-the-counter medications such as aspirin and ibuprofen. The pain was constant and she noticed she was most comfortable in positions in which her head was supported. Over-the-counter medications did not help much and she sought help from her primary care physician. She was given various pain medications. Because her head tilted toward the left shoulder and her left shoulder was elevated, her doctor prescribed physical therapy for muscular strain. Neither the medications nor the physical therapy helped the pain she felt in her neck, head, and left shoulder. She developed stomach problems due to the pain medications. Because of the pain, she was unable to continue working and lost her job in a department store. She became depressed over this and mentioned it to her doctor, who referred her to a psychiatrist. The psychiatrist gave her antidepressant medication and, although her mood improved, the pain in her neck did not. She then was referred to a pain specialist who gave her nerve block injections and even destroyed one of the nerves thought to be causing her pain. The pain continued. She finally was diagnosed with CD when she was referred to a neurologist for treatment of her continuing headaches.

Whether a neurologist provides more advanced treatment for CD depends on the concentration of his or her practice. Therefore, a neurologist will sometimes refer patients who do not respond well to treatment, or those who have severe or complicated cases, to a subspecialist in the field of movement disorders. Neurology clinics specializing in movement disorders are mostly found at major university medical centers, although some neurologists specializing in movement disorders practice at private medical centers, in private groups, or independently in the community.

The neurologist will try to ascertain the presence of factors in your medical history known to cause movement disorders. If other causes of dystonia are not found during the interview, the physician should suspect the presence of an idiopathic movement disorder and will then examine you thoroughly. He may first want to establish the presence of over-contracting or spasming muscles in the neck by looking carefully for their bulging and also by feeling the relative firmness or flaccidity of various muscles. Experienced physicians can often tell by carefully observing head position and direction of tremor movement, and by sense of touch, exactly which particular neck muscles are primarily involved in the CD.

The physician will usually perform a more generalized neurologic exam to look for coexisting conditions or dystonic involvement of other body parts. He may look for problems in memory and cognitive abilities, disorders affecting the pyramidal motor system, spinal cord problems, and dystonia affecting any of the limbs, face, eye closure muscles, or voice. He may order laboratory tests to screen for some of the medical disorders discussed previously that can produce dystonia.

Depending on the presence of certain factors in your medical history or findings on the physical exam, the physician may order X-ray study, CT scan, or MRI of the neck to ascertain the presence of an orthopedic abnormality in the cervical spine. A brain imaging study, usually an MRI, may be indicated if there is a history of stroke or head trauma. As previously discussed, the basal ganglia abnormalities that produce CD are not visible on MRI. Once other conditions are eliminated by history, physical examination, and any indicated tests, the definitive diagnosis of idiopathic CD may be made.

OTHER CERVICAL CONDITIONS

Spasmodic torticollis, the neurological movement disorder, needs to be distinguished from a number of other neck conditions, some of which produce abnormal posture.

Tension Cervicalgia

The most common condition confused with CD is sometimes called "wry neck," although this term has been loosely used for a variety of conditions, including CD. Wry neck is usually a result of an acute neck muscle spasm or strain that produces pain. Nearly everyone at some time has awoken one morning with a new neck pain, or a "crick" in the neck. A person so affected may *intentionally* hold his or her head in a position so as to minimize the pain, or may be reluctant to turn the head normally to look in a different direction. Instead, he or she may turn his or her entire body to look in a particular direction, giving the appearance of a "stiff" neck. We prefer to use the term "tension cervicalgia" to refer to this condition. We prefer not to use the term "wry neck" at all, since its meaning is ambiguous. Tension cervicalgia usually abates with conservative treatments such as stretching, massage, posture correction, and simple analgesics.

Orthopedic Conditions

CD is a neurologic disorder, with the pathological process occurring mainly in the motor part of the brain. A number of muscular and skeletal conditions may resemble CD. Some children are born with one or more neck muscles shortened, otherwise poorly formed, or missing altogether, creating a tethering effect that results in malposition of the head and a restricted range of neck motion. Another musculoskeletal condition is *atlanto-axial dislocation,* a slippage of the top two bones of the vertebral column, which occurs as a result of physical injury. These muscular and skeletal conditions fall under the realm of orthopedics rather than neurology. They can mimic the appearance of CD, but are not caused by abnormal signals from the CNS producing dystonic contractions of a set of muscles. Orthopedic conditions will not respond to the treatments used for neurologic CD; they are usually treated with physical therapy, splints, collars, or surgery. There is extensive literature on various forms of orthopedic torticollis affecting infants and young children, but these conditions will not be discussed in this book.

Drug-Induced Conditions

Drug-induced conditions caused by medicines used to treat nausea and vomiting, and certain psychiatric medicines called *neuroleptics* or *antipsychotics* can result in tardive dyskinesia or dystonia that closely resembles CD and persists after the medication has been stopped. This is probably the reason that torticollis is often perceived as a psychiatric condition. It should be stressed that the tardive dyskinesia is not a result of the psychiatric illness, but a complication of the medications used to treat it. Drug-induced movement disorders are discussed in more detail in Chapter 4.

TREATMENT OF CERVICAL DYSTONIA

Chemodenervation

Chemodenervation with botulinum toxin has been discussed previously in Chapter 11. We will discuss here only some of its unique features in the treatment of CD.

The effectiveness of botulinum toxin in any person with dystonia depends on the severity of his condition. Botulinum toxin never fully restores the natural resting position. For our own patients, our goal is to improve head position by 50% to 70%, and we select muscles and injection doses according to this goal. Fortunately, botulinum toxin is as effective, if not more effective, in ameliorating the pain component of CD as it is in improving head position. This is often more important to the person suffering from CD.

Some patients expect that their CD will continue to improve progressively with each successive treatment until the condition is completely resolved. This is unfortunately not the case. Symptoms return as the effect of botulinum toxin wears off. For instance, suppose a patient with a rotational torticollis of 60 degrees receives chemodenervation treatment and that the rotation subsequently improves to 30 degrees. As the toxin's effect wears off over time, the patient's head will slowly drift back approximately to the original 60 degrees of rotation. Subsequent chemodenervation treatments should have about the same effect as the first one, improving the rotation to approximately 30 degrees. Subsequent treatments will not progressively improve rotation until neutral position is reached.

A few patients have even noticed that the results from their first chemodenervation were the best, and that subsequent treatments did not produce the same degree of improvement. This phenomenon has many explanations, which may vary from individual to individual. There are many muscles participating in the pulling of CD and we treat only the largest and most accessible muscles. Many smaller muscles are therefore left untreated. Therefore, even in the best scenario, some residual head pulling persists. After some length of time, uninjected muscles, often smaller and deeper in the neck, may take over the lead, pulling the head back to its abnormal set point.

We have seen, during neck surgery on some of our patients for whom chemodenervation treatments had become ineffective over time, that some of these deep, normally small muscles had become enlarged from the involuntary exercise. Our inability to identify such muscles (prior to surgery), or the inability to inject them without substantial risk to the patient, may account for the diminished effectiveness of subsequent chemodenervation treatments in some patients. However, an experienced physician may be able to cope with this problem by varying the injection technique to target these previously untreated muscles.

Difficulty with holding the head upright may occur if larger doses are required for severe CD cases. The toxin may also spread from the point of injection through tissues of the neck to the larynx, or voice box. The usual result is mild swallowing difficulty or hoarseness of the voice, requiring a soft or pureed diet for several days. Rarely, breathing difficulties can occur. Most side effects resolve over days or weeks. There is no known permanent impairment from botulinum toxin injection. Botulinum toxin injection for chemodenervation is now a principal treatment for CD, and is recommended by the American Academy of Neurology and the National Institutes of Health.

Surgical Treatment

In order to discuss surgical treatment, we will have to further discuss the anatomy of the neck. The cervical spine is depicted in Figure 1. Each vertebra of the spine is shaped like a ring, with a hole in the middle. When they are stacked together to form the cervical spine, the holes form the *central spinal canal*, through which runs the spinal cord (Figure 17). At each vertebral level, the spinal cord gives off a pair of right and left nerve roots that contain the outflow axons of neurons of the motor system. The nerve roots exit the cervical spine through gaps between the vertebrae called *foramina*. The roots

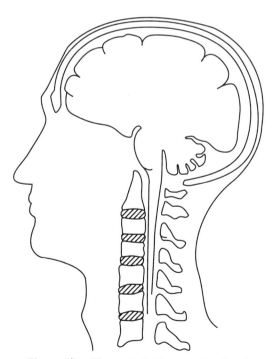

Figure 17 *The cervical spine and spinal cord.*

may merge with each other. Either before or after merging, they branch into motor nerves that terminate in various muscles. One single nerve root may supply signals to a number of muscles, but each muscle receives its signals mainly through one single terminal motor nerve branch.

Peripheral Surgery

The spinal nerve roots are fairly easy for a surgeon to locate at the point where they exit between the vertebrae of the cervical spine. One easy way to stop overactive agonist muscles would be to cut those nerve roots that supply them, a procedure known as *rhizotomy* (Figure 18).

There are drawbacks to such an approach, however. Since one root supplies several muscles, many more than just the targeted agonists would become severely weakened or paralyzed, causing excessive neck weakness. Since the surgery is permanent, there would be no way to reverse this weakness. Although there are variants of

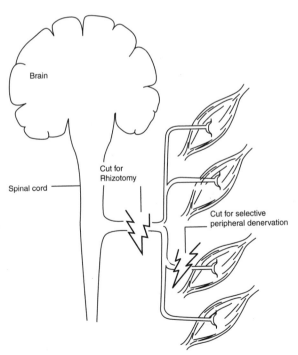

Figure 18 *Surgical sites for rhizotomy and selective peripheral denervation.*

rhizotomy that involve only partial cutting of a nerve root, this procedure has largely been superseded by a technique known as *selective peripheral denervation.*

The technique of selective peripheral denervation was developed in the 1970s by Dr. Claude Betrand. It requires somewhat more finesse than the standard rhizotomy described above. In this procedure, a surgeon must locate motor nerve branches supplying the targeted agonist muscles, follow them to their termination point in the muscle, and cut them just at that point (Figure 18). Selective peripheral denervation is a highly specialized procedure; it should be performed by an experienced neurosurgeon in conjunction with a movement disorders specialist.

The muscles to be targeted must be carefully selected prior to the surgery. Sometimes, the best muscles to target are difficult to identify, even for an experienced movement disorders specialist using EMG guidance before and during the surgery. Our strategy, for some of our more complex patients, has been to first perform a partial operation, targeting only those muscles that are obviously involved. We then allow the patient to recover out of the hospital, after which we carefully reassess him to select target muscles for a second surgery. The goal is to abolish the abnormal contraction in most of the muscles producing the unwanted movement, while preserving nerve connections to adjacent normally acting muscles. Selective peripheral denervation works best for patients with rotational torticollis and least for patients with retrocollis. Physical therapy is required to recover the full range of motion of the neck following surgery.

Adverse effects from surgery include a permanent weakness of adjacent neck muscles that causes difficulty in holding up the head or in swallowing. Rarely, weakness of the diaphragm can occur, causing a breathing impairment, because the nerve that controls this muscle passes close to some target muscles. Fortunately, we have been able to substantially reduce the occurrence of these adverse effects in recent years by refinements in surgical technique. For instance, we use an electrical nerve stimulation technique that allows us to identify and cut a nerve at a point just before it enters the target muscle, well after it has already given off branches to adjacent muscles, such as those involved in swallowing. Despite all refinements, however, there are anatomic and physiologic variations among patients, and adverse events may still occur.

Another surgical procedure is called *myotomy*. Myotomy involves the cutting or removal of portions of the overactive agonist muscles. Because of the greater amount of tissue trauma from this procedure, internal scar tissue may form and adhere to adjacent muscles and ligaments, limiting the range of neck motion or causing pain. Although myotomy may still be applied in certain cases, selective peripheral denervation is more appropriate when the muscle involved can be exactly identified.

Brain Surgery

The techniques of thallamotomy, pallidotomy, and deep brain stimulator implantation have already been discussed in detail. While applicable to generalized dystonia, these have so far not been as effective for cervical dystonia. Among these techniques, DBS has shown limited success, and holds the most promise for future application to cervical dystonia if the correct basal ganglia target for the stimulator wire can be found.

Spine Surgery

The authors have seen a small number of patients who had received cervical spine fusion surgery for the treatment of CD. Basically, this involves the harvesting of pieces of shaved bone from other parts of the body, then grafting them into place as bridges across adjacent cervical vertebral bones. The grafted pieces of bone fuse into place, locking adjacent vertebrae together into a rigid, unbendable column. This may seem like a logical way to keep the head straight, but think about this: the abnormally contracting muscles will continue to exert their pulling force. The difference is that they will now exert tension and torsion forces on joints that cannot bend or give way. In our experience, this creates worse bone and muscle pain than before. In such patients, pain may become so severe that they are forced to use narcotics on a chronic basis. We have attempted to treat such patients by chemodenervation with botulinum toxin injections or with selective peripheral denervation. However, these two treatments often fail to relieve pain symptoms in patients who have had spinal fusion. The reason for this is that not every single muscle involved in the CD can be targeted for injection or denervation, and these leftover secondary muscles continue to exert a small pulling force. Even this small residual pulling force is enough to produce pain when it is applied against a rigid, unyielding spinal column. Spinal fusion surgery may be appropriate for patients who suffer from *orthopedic* causes of torticollis, but it is not appropriate for patients who have CD, the *neurologic* movement disorder. In our experience, we have never found spinal fusion surgery to have benefited any CD patients who have had it done. It is simply not helpful, and may be harmful.

WHO WILL BENEFIT FROM SURGERY?

All surgical procedures carry the risk of producing excessive weakness or paralysis, causing infection or internal bleeding, complications of anesthesia, or simply not being effective. In light of these considerations, how are candidates for surgery selected from among CD patients? Simply put, all nonsurgical treatments are attempted first. Surgery is never considered as a first-line or early treatment, even in fairly severe cases, because a few may resolve spontaneously, given time. Additionally, the specific muscles involved at the beginning may change over time. Some muscles may stop contracting and new ones may become involved. The proper muscles to target may not become obvious until the disorder stabilizes. Chemodenervation with botulinum toxin remains the mainstay of treatment for CD, supplemented by oral medications and pain management. As discussed previously, some patients may develop resistance to botulinum toxin after years of repeated injections. Those patients for whom chemodenervation is no longer effective may be considered for surgery. Among those patients, surgery works best for those with rotational torticollis, and less well for those who predominantly have retrocollis or anterocollis. Other factors may influence a patient's suitability for surgery. The coexistence of medical conditions such as heart disease, diabetes, lung or breathing problems, or blood clotting abnormalities will add to the risk of adverse outcomes from surgery. Selective peripheral denervation or DBS are becoming the procedure of choice for those patients who are appropriate candidates for surgery. Note that, as opposed to *surgical* denervation, the injection of phenol or botulinum toxin achieves a *chemical* denervation. Chemodenervation with botulinum toxin is not permanent, but destructive surgery is. Also, surgery of any kind rarely completely cures CD. Peripheral surgeries on the nerves and muscles do not alter the abnormality in the extrapyramidal system of the brain. The brain may recruit adjacent muscles, usually smaller and often not previously involved in the CD, into activity in order to bring the head back to its abnormal set point. Patients who undergo surgery do not usually become free from the need for continued treatment. Many of them must continue receiving botulinum toxin injections and/or medications. All of the factors discussed above must be considered together in selecting any one patient for surgery.

Physical Therapy

If available, physical therapy by an experienced therapist may improve pain symptoms. The goals of physical therapy include bringing the head position back toward normal, increasing the range of motion, and decreasing pain, thereby increasing functional ability. The physical therapist may employ a variety of techniques to achieve these goals. Primarily, he will gently move the neck through its range of motion, stretching the spasming agonist muscles. He may take advantage of the effect of geste antagoniste, stimulating the skin by gentle stroking or by applying ice to decrease the contraction of agonists during neck maneuvers. For some patients, gentle neck traction using a mechanical device may alleviate pain. Physical therapy techniques such as ultrasound or diathermy also may help with pain.

Massage

While it is used extensively by some of our patients and is a fairly effective treatment for tension cervicalgia, local massage tends to have mixed results in CD. While it almost always feels good while being performed, pain control is very short-lived. In some patients, massage, especially deep massage, aggravates the spasms and contractions of agonist muscles. As a result, pain may actually *increase* following massage. However, we have found that an acupressure type treatment, in which the point of an elbow is applied to a spasming trapezius muscle, or to muscles in the back of the neck, is often beneficial. Pressure should not be applied to the sternocleidomastoid muscle, which runs along the front and side of the neck, since doing so is ineffective and may even cause injury. Overall, we have found that properly applied acupressure is a most economical and effective pain relief measure with very low risk or side effects, and it may be performed at home by a spouse or family member.

Chiropractic

Chiropractic manipulation of the neck is generally safe. It is dangerous only in a cervical spine that has been fractured, that has an unstable dislocation of one or more vertebrae, or that has arthritic changes that may predispose to damaging an important artery during manipulation, resulting in a stroke. Other than in these situations, which most chiropractors will exclude by examination and X-rays, chiropractic intervention carries minimal risk, especially with the modern safer neck manipulation techniques in wide use today. However, we find that the vocabulary employed in the chiropractic realm is not quite the same as ours. Torticollis, as diagnosed by a chiropractor, may not be exactly the same condition as the neurologic movement disorder we are discussing in this book. Additionally, treatments and techniques vary widely among chiropractors, and it is impossible for us to comment on the benefit any one patient may experience by visiting an individual chiropractor. Overall, in the medical literature, chiropractic manipulation has not been shown to be effective in alleviating either the abnormal neck posture or the pain associated with neurologic CD.

Cervical Collars

We are aware of rare patients who are able to use collars to ease their performance in specific situations. For instance, one of our patients wraps a soft collar about her neck while driving. The rubbing of the soft foam rubber against her skin provides a *geste antagoniste* that aids her in looking forward down the road. However, she does not use the collar at most other times. Cervical collars may provide a feeling of temporary relief from CD, however, they may also cause harm. Cervical collars are intended for short-term use, and CD is usually a chronic (long-term) problem. Use of a cervical collar over a period of months may lead to weakening of the neck musculature—all muscles, not just those that are overactive. Cervical collars, especially the hard collars, rub against the back of the neck and can induce muscle spasms. Uncontrolled head motion may even cause enough rubbing against the collar to break or ulcerate the skin, especially in older patients. These effects can make the torticollis worse or increase the pain. Finally, hard collars may increase the chance of neck injury; a dislocation of the spinal bones can result from falling down the wrong way while wearing a hard cervical collar. For these reasons, we rarely recommend cervical collars in the treatment of CD.

Miscellaneous

Other forms of treatment may also be helpful. Occupational therapy can help with stress management, mobility, energy conservation, and the use of adaptive equipment. Psychological counseling may help patients to understand the nature of their pain and the effects it can have on them, and techniques for coping with chronic pain can be learned. Hypnosis, while not harmful, has not been found to be useful, because CD is not primarily a psychiatric disorder. Biofeedback, acupuncture, and acupressure are alternative treatments that may aid in pain management. A transepidermal nerve stimulator unit, a wearable device that delivers low-level tingling electrical stimulation to the skin, can provide temporary pain relief. Your doctor may refer you to a physical therapy facility, a pain management clinic, or a practitioner who specializes in these various interventions.

14

Coping

Our patients who are diagnosed with dystonia share many of the responses of patients diagnosed with any chronic disease. They wonder how the disorder will affect their employment or professional lives, and how it will affect their personal and sexual relationships.

Dystonia is a very noticeable medical disorder. When we think of those chronic neurologic illnesses that are perceived by our patients as creating a social stigma, few are as immediately obvious to casual observers as dystonia. This is especially true of cervical dystonia, which affects the head and neck, and other dystonias that affect the facial muscles. Our face, head, and neck are the most visible parts of our bodies, and it is with these that we do most of our communicating. Not only our verbal output, but also our facial expressions and head movements, are continuously used—overtly and subtly—to interact with other people. Dystonia disrupts this communication in a very obvious way, especially if the dystonia also involves facial and neck muscles. It is impossible to hide. Add to this the fact that people with dystonia are sometimes perceived as having an underlying psychiatric condition, and you can see that this disorder can severely impair social interactions.

In our years of treating patients with dystonia and other disabling neurologic conditions including paraplegia, Parkinson disease, and stroke, we have seen these common initial reactions to becoming disabled or diagnosed with an incurable condition. Self-consciousness and social embarrassment can cause patients to become socially disengaged, give up public activities, and may become as disabling as the physical symptoms of the disease. Social embarrassment is one of the "hidden symptoms" of dystonia. Some patients become clinically depressed, requiring treatment for this condition as well.

We have found, however, that no matter how severe the initial reactions, patient optimism seems to win out over feelings of despair. The course generally takes 1 to 2 years from the time of occurrence or diagnosis. Those who persevere through this phase become surprisingly well adapted to their new state of health and ability. Social embarrassment diminishes greatly and, even if it persists, we rarely see patients who allow it to impede them in pursuing an active life socially or professionally. Many look back on the initial phase of their illness and wonder why their despair or embarrassment was so great at the time.

What advice do we have for those newly diagnosed with dystonia? Simply this: persevere. Be patient but persistent as you go through the medical system. Specialists experienced in treating your condition may be few in your location, but once under their management, you will find significant relief with current treatment options. Unlike some neurologic disorders, dystonia is not an inexorably disabling condition. Your pain and your outward symptoms will almost certainly improve with medical management, and your self-confidence and outlook will do likewise.

We advocate joining a patient support group, some of which are listed in the resources section of this book. Travel to one of their national, regional, or local meetings to share your experiences, management strategies, and tips for managing routine daily activities with other dystonia sufferers. If depression or psychological distress becomes problematic, do not disregard this aspect of your disorder. Seek evaluation with a psychiatrist, psychological counsellor, or other professional.

Maintaining optimal health is the best way to cope with a chronic disorder such as dystonia. A healthy diet and regular cardiovascular exercise are important to achieve this goal. No vitamins, minerals, or special diets have proved to be beneficial specifically for dystonia. Stimulants such as caffeine and nicotine may transiently aggravate dystonia symptoms; however, there is no evidence that these substances cause permanent worsening. Although alcohol can have some muscle relaxing effects and briefly improves a few movement disorders, its use is not recommended as a treatment for dystonia.

Exercise is an important part of maintaining health, but there are a few things you should keep in mind if you have dystonia. It is important to maintain as much flexibility as possible. Gentle stretching exercises are recommended. You should avoid sudden manipulations or extremes of movement with respect to your neck and spine. The concept of "no pain, no gain" does not apply here; you should let pain be your indicator to quit an exercise. Otherwise, judicious aerobic exercise is good for your cardiovascular system and maintaining optimal health. For the most part, stretching and strengthening exercises for the back and limbs can be found in many general books on yoga, calesthenics, and other exercise. The following chapter contains a number of stretching and strengthening exercises that were developed specifically for cervical dystonia sufferers.

Our patients have similar advice, as you will have seen throughout the book. One patient with cervical dystonia offered the following tips to living well with dystonia:

- Take the time to research and find out who in your area treats the disorder.
- Don't take "no" for an answer from the insurance company.
- Accept the diagnosis and adjust your life appropriately; life goes on after diagnosis.
- Seek out a support group.
- Remember that you have nothing to be ashamed of.
- Modify activities in a way that reduces strain.
- Learn to pace yourself.
- Get out in public and do the things that you enjoy; being active is important both physically and mentally.
- Have a positive attitude about your disorder, and so will others.
- Journaling sometimes helps.
- Don't despair; get out there in the world, be a productive member of society, and get involved.

15

Rehabilitation Exercises

SPECIFIC EXERCISES YOU CAN DO AT HOME

This chapter describes some exercises that you can perform on your own. They are specific for the treatment of cervical dystonia (CD) and any other dystonia that affects neck muscles. Involvement of neck muscles often causes the most pain and discomfort among dystonia patients. These exercises and are designed to accomplish two major goals:

1. Stretch and relax the overactive muscles that are in spasm (*agonists*).
2. Strengthen the muscles that can oppose the torticollis and bring the head position back to neutral (*antagonists*).

The exercises in this chapter are designed to be used in conjunction with medical treatments such as oral medications, chemodenervation injections, physical therapy, and pain management interventions.

In general, you will be applying the stretching exercises to the overactive agonist muscles in conjunction with chemodenervation. As the overactive muscles are weakened by chemodenervation, they will be easier to stretch using the above exercises. As they relax and their pulling force diminishes, it will become easier to perform strengthening exercises on the opposing antagonist muscles. The exercises appropriate for you will depend upon the muscles involved in your particular case of CD. Ask your treating physician to specify which of your muscles are acting as agonists. In general, these are the ones that are being injected with botulinum toxin, and you should practice those stretching exercises specific for them. Also ask your physician which antagonist muscles he would recommend for strengthening. In most cases, these will be the muscles that correspond to the agonists on the opposite side of your neck, but additional antagonists may need strengthening as well. If you have a physical therapist, he or she may be able to help in selecting the particular muscles and exercises that are appropriate for you.

The exercises have been designed to be performed with a bare minimum of easily obtained equipment. With a few modifications, they can be performed in almost any setting, at home or at work. All of the exercises described are to be performed slowly—you should perform all of them in slow motion. If any movement produces pain, you should stop and seek further advice from your doctor.

STRETCHING EXERCISES

The first exercises that follow are simple stretches. Many of the following stretching exercises can be done in the standing or seated position. Most require some type of suitable handhold. In the standing position, the height of the handhold should be about the mid-thigh level, close to where the hand rests naturally. A suitable object to grasp might be a heavy table or desk. In the seated position, a sturdy chair with a suitable leg or cross bar should suffice. For some exercises requiring a handhold in front of you, the front edge of the seat may be grasped. Use a stable chair with a backrest and without wheels. The illustrations depict a common type of inexpensive metal folding chair available at most office or home warehouse stores.

Exercise 1: Splenius Capitis, Levator Scapuli, and Others

This exercise is designed to stretch and relax the muscles that run down the back of your neck on either side of your neck bones, as well as the muscles that connect these bones to your shoulder blades. It may be useful for individuals who have a component of rotational torticollis plus retrocollis (see Chapter 13, Figure 16). It is performed in a seated position on a chair that allows you to grasp and hold underneath (Figure 1). Alternatively, it can be performed in the standing position next to an object that has a handhold at approximately the mid-thigh level. We will illustrate stretching for the left-sided muscles. The entire procedure may be reversed if you require stretching of the right-sided muscles.

Grasp the handhold with your left hand. Slowly lean your body forward and toward the right side, and at the same time allow your left shoulder to relax and be pulled downward while keeping your grip on the handhold. You may feel a pulling or stretching sensation deep in your shoulder muscles. Next, turn your head about 45 degrees toward the right, then tilt your head in a direction away from your left arm. As you do this, feel the stretch in the muscles of your shoulder and the back of your neck on the left side. Hold this position for 30 seconds. You may feel the sensation of stretch begin to subside.

At this point, you may actually be able to stretch a little further. To make the stretch even more effective, reach over the top of your head with your right hand and gently help pull along the direction of the stretch (Figure 2). Hold this position for another 10 seconds, then slowly release and relax.

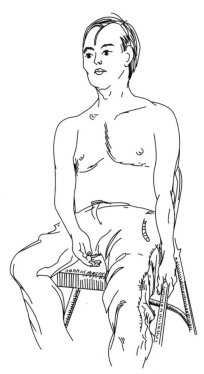

Figure 1   *Slowly lean your body forward and towards the right. Relax your left shoulder, allowing it to be pulled downward. Rotate your head 45 degrees to the right, and then tilt your head away from your left arm. Hold for 30 seconds.*

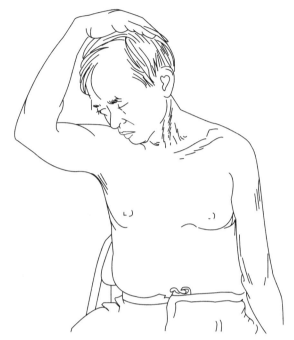

Figure 2   *Reach over the top of your head with your right hand and gently pull your head in the direction of the stretch. Hold for 10 seconds, then slowly release and relax.*

Exercise 2: Sternocleidomastoid on One Side

This next exercise is intended to provide stretch to one of the major muscles that runs diagonally across the front and side of the neck and has attachments at the collar bone and the back of the skull. Known as the sternocleidomastoid (SCM), this is one of the muscles most frequently involved in CD. The left SCM's normal action is to rotate the head toward the right while also tucking the chin downward to the chest (see Chapter 13, Figure 6). The movements in this particular exercise are somewhat complex, and will require some patience and practice to be performed correctly. We will illustrate stretching for the left SCM. The entire procedure may be reversed if you require stretching of the right SCM. In order to stretch the left SCM, begin in a seated or standing position. Grasp the handhold behind or underneath you with your left hand (Figure 3). Now lean your body slightly so that your left shoulder is pulled downward. If you relax your shoulder, you will find that your collarbone is pulled downward. Now slowly rotate your head toward the left side (the side being stretched).

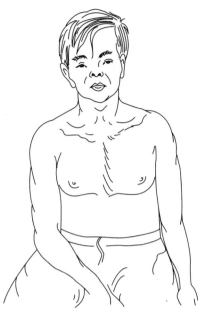

Figure 3   *Lean your body slightly to pull your left shoulder downward. Slowly rotate your head towards the left side as far as it can comfortably go.*

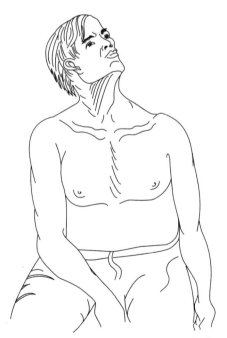

Figure 4   *Tilt your head back so that your chin moves towards the ceiling and then down towards your right shoulder as far as it will comfortably go. Hold for 30 seconds.*

Once your head has been rotated as far as it can comfortably go, begin tilting your head backward so that your chin moves toward the ceiling. Now tilt your head slightly so that your right ear moves closer to your right shoulder (Figure 4). As you do this, you may feel a stretching sensation from your left collarbone to the side of neck. Hold at the point you feel stretch but not pain. After 30 seconds, the feeling of stretch may begin to subside. At this point, you may increase the stretch a little further by cupping the fingers of your left hand around your chin and slowly and gently pushing upwards. As always, stop if you feel pain. Hold this position for 10 more seconds, then slowly release and relax.

Exercise 3: Sternocleidomastoid on Both Sides

The next exercise is a simple alternative stretch for the SCM that stretches both sides at once, and may be useful for individuals with anterocollis (see Chapter 13, Figure 2). This is best done in a seated position in a chair with some support for the back (Figure 5). Simply grasp a handhold underneath you with one or both hands. Allow

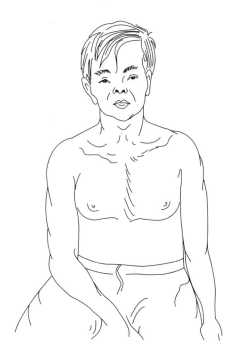

Figure 5   *Slowly lean backwards, relaxing your shoulders, to pull your shoulders and collarbone downward. Keep your head facing directly forward!*

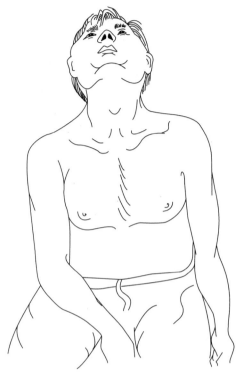

Figure 6 *Slowly tilt your head back so that your chin is pointing towards the ceiling. Keep your shoulders relaxed and downward. Hold for 30 seconds, then slowly release and relax.*

your shoulder muscles to relax, pulling down your collarbones. Keep your head in the neutral position facing directly ahead! Now, slowly tilt your head backward so that your chin moves toward the ceiling (Figure 6). You should feel a stretching sensation in the front and side of your neck. Do not hunch up your shoulders; allow them to relax and be pulled downward. Hold at the point where you feel stretch but not unusual pain. Hold this position for 30 seconds, then slowly release and relax.

Exercise 4: Trapezius, Levator Scapuli, Sternocleidomastoid, and Scalenes

The next exercise is intended to provide stretch for the muscles that lift the shoulder upwards and tilt the head directly sideways, mainly the trapezius and levator scapuli, but also the scalenes and

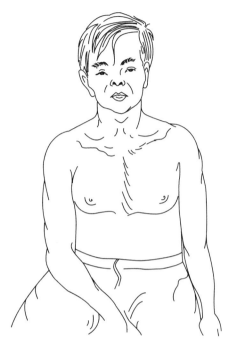

Figure 7   *Lean your body to the right while relaxing your shoulder muscles, allowing your shoulder to be pulled down. Tilt your head sideways and to the right. Hold for 30 seconds.*

SCM. This exercise is useful for persons who have lateralcollis (see Chapter 13, Figure 5). We have selected the left-sided muscles for illustration. The entire procedure may be reversed if you require stretching of the right-sided muscles. Starting from the seated or standing position, grasp a handhold beside you with your left hand (Figure 7). Lean your body to the right while relaxing your shoulder muscles and allowing your shoulder to be pulled downward. Now, tilt your head sideways to the right. You may feel a stretching sensation from the shoulder to the side of the neck. Hold this position for 30 seconds. You may feel the sensation of stretching begin to subside. At this point, you can increase the stretch a little further by placing your right hand over the top of your head and slowly and gently pulling to the right (Figure 8). Stop if you feel any unusual pain. Hold this position for another 10 seconds, then slowly release and relax.

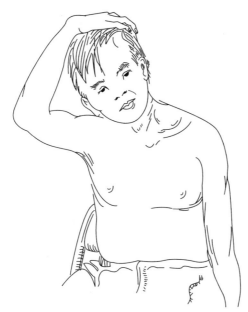

Figure 8 *Place your right hand over the top of your head and pull slowly and gently to the right. Hold for another 10 seconds, and then release and relax.*

Exercise 5: Splenius Capitis

The next exercise is intended to provide stretch to several muscles in the back of the neck, mainly the splenius capitis (SC). This muscle starts at the neck bones and runs diagonally upward and outward to the base of the skull. The normal action of the right SC is to pull the head backwards and rotate it slightly to the right side (similar to Chapter 13, Figure 13). This exercise is similar to Exercise 1, but is more specific for the SC. We will illustrate stretching for the right SC. The entire procedure may be reversed if you require stretching of your left SC. To stretch the right SC, start in the seated or standing position. First rotate your head toward the left, then tilt your head downward, tucking your chin toward your chest (Figure 9). You may begin feeling a stretching sensation in the back of your neck, on one or both sides. Hold this position for 30 seconds. You may feel the stretching sensation begin to subside. At this point, you may increase the stretch a little further by placing your fingers against the side of your chin and gently pushing to rotate your chin toward your left shoulder (Figure 10). Hold this position for another 10 seconds, then slowly release and relax.

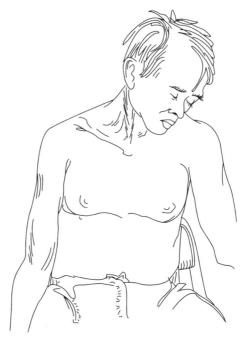

Figure 9   *Rotate your head towards the left, then tilt it downward, trucking your chin into your chest. Hold for 30 seconds. Feel the stretch in the back of your neck.*

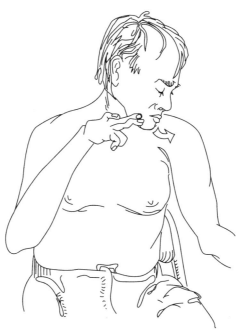

Figure 10   *Place two fingers against the side of your chin and gently push your chin towards your left shoulder. Hold for 10 seconds, and then slowly release and relax.*

STRENGTHENING EXERCISES

The next set of exercises is designed to strengthen the antagonist muscles. Strengthening these muscles can help to bring your head back to the neutral position. To strengthen any muscle, it is necessary to use it to exert a force against resistance. Thus, to perform these exercises, you will need a suitable object against which to push. A pillow-sized block of soft foam rubber works best and may be obtained from a medical supply store or pharmacy. A larger, thick block of foam is best. Suitable thicker foam pillows may also be found in department and bedding stores. Most of the following exercises can be modified for performance in the sitting, standing, or lying position. In most cases, resistance supplied by an opposing hand or fingers can be substituted for the foam block or pillow, allowing the exercises to be performed in almost any situation. If you are not able to perform an exercise against resistance, try the movement by itself at first, using no type of resistance.

Exercise 6: Sternocleidomastoid on One Side

This exercise is designed to strengthen the SCM muscle on one side. Overactivity of the *right* SCM produces rotational torticollis toward the *left* (Figure 11), in which case strengthening of the *left* SCM is required. This entire procedure may be reversed if you require strengthening of your right SCM. To strengthen the left SCM, start in a seated position parallel to a wall. Your right shoulder should just barely touch the wall. Place the foam block on top of your right shoulder flush with the wall (Figure 12). Place the side of your face snugly against the block. Now turn your head slowly as if looking to your right. Rotate your head until you are pressing as hard as you comfortably can (Figure 13). Hold for 30 seconds, then release and relax. Repeat this exercise three to five times per exercise session. Increase as tolerated. Some people may only be able to perform this exercise without a pillow; resistance provided by placing a hand on the side of the face may suffice. Others may not be able to push against a resistance at all.

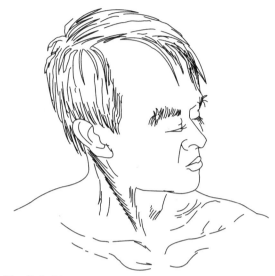

Figure 11   *Left-side rotational torticollis caused by overactivity in the right sternocleidomastoid.*

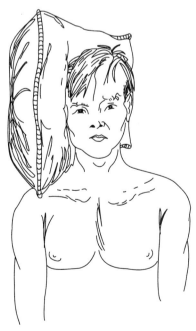

Figure 12   *Place the foam block on top of your right shoulder, flush with the wall.*

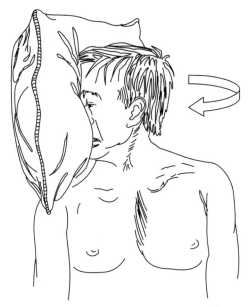

Figure 13 *Turn your head to the right slowly, rotating it until you are pressing as hard as you can. Hold this position for 30 seconds, and then release and relax. Repeat three to five times.*

Exercise 7: Trapezius and Levator Scapuli

The next exercise is intended to strengthen the muscles that elevate the shoulder and shoulder blade, mainly the trapezius and the levator scapuli. We have selected the left-sided muscles for illustration. The entire procedure may be reversed if you require strengthening of the right-sided muscles. To strengthen the left-sided muscles, start in the seated or standing position. Grasp a handhold beside you with your left hand. Now slowly shrug your left shoulder without moving your head (Figure 14). Remember that the pulling should be done with your shoulder shrug only. Try to keep your arm straight and do not try to lift by bending your arm at the elbow. Pull with your shoulder muscles as hard as you comfortably can, hold for 30 seconds, then slowly release and relax. Repeat this exercise three to five times per exercise session. Increase as tolerated to a maximum of 12 repetitions.

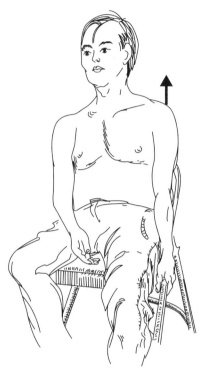

Figure 14 *Slowly shrug your left shoulder, keeping your head still. Pull your muscles up as hard as you comfortably can. Hold for 30 seconds. Repeat three to five times.*

Exercise 8: Splenius Capitis and Others on One Side

This exercise is designed to strengthen the muscles that lie along the back of the neck on either side of the neck bones. These include the diagonally running SC and other deeper muscles. The left SC tilts the head backward and turns the chin slightly toward the left. Movement produced mainly by the left SC is depicted in Chapter 13, Figure 16. This person requires strengthening of the right-sided SC (he or she should also strengthen the left SCM). We have selected the right SC for illustration. The entire procedure may be reversed if you require strengthening of your left SC. To strengthen your right SC, start the exercise lying on your back with the foam pillow underneath your head (Figure 15). Rotate your head approximately 45 degrees to the right. Now tilt your head backwards, pushing into the foam pillow (Figure 16). Try to push against the block with the part

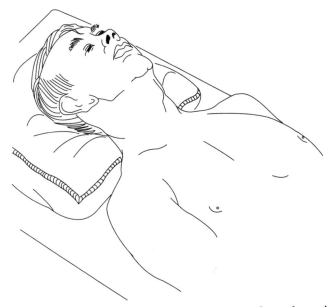

Figure 15 *Lie on your back and place a foam pillow underneath your head.*

of your head immediately behind and above your right ear. Push as hard as you comfortably can, hold for 10 seconds, then slowly release and relax. Repeat this exercise three to five times per exercise session. Increase as tolerated, to a maximum of 12 repetitions.

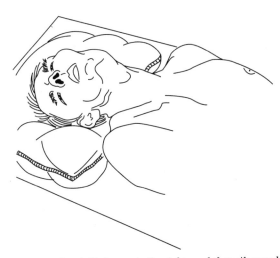

Figure 16 *Rotate your head 45 degrees to the right, and then tilt your head backwards into the foam block. Push as hard as you comfortably can. Hold for 10 seconds, then slowly release and relax. Repeat three to five times.*

Exercise 9: Sternocleidomastoids on Both Sides

This is an alternative exercise that can be used if both the right and left SCM muscles need to be strengthened. It may be useful for individuals with retrocollis (see Chapter 13, Figure 3). Start by lying flat on your back (Figure 17). Now lift your head straight upwards, tilting your chin slightly toward your chest. If desired, push against your forehead with two fingers as shown to provide resistance (Figure 18).

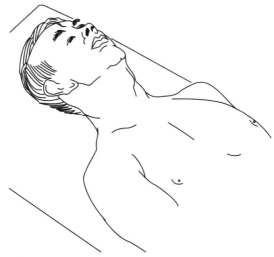

Figure 17 *Lie flat on your back and lift your head straight up, tilting your chin slightly towards your chest.*

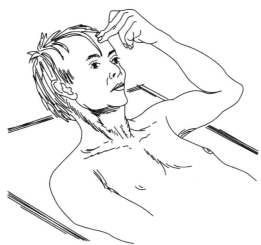

Figure 18 *Using two fingers, push down against your forehead as you continue to lift and tilt. Hold for 10 seconds, and then slowly release and relax. Repeat three to five times.*

Hold this position for 10 seconds, then slowly release and relax. Repeat this exercise three to five times per exercise session. Increase as tolerated, to a maximum of 12 repetitions.

Exercise 10: Sternocleidomastoid, Trapezius, Levator Scapuli, and Scalenes

This exercise is designed to strengthen the muscles that tilt the head sideways and elevate the shoulder, including the SCM, trapezius, and levator scapuli. The individual shown in Figure 10 has lateral-collis produced by overactivity of left-sided muscles, and requires strengthening on the right. We have selected the right sided muscles for illustration. The entire procedure may be reversed if you require strengthening of your left-sided muscles. To strengthen the right-sided muscles, begin in the seated position on a chair with your right shoulder touching the wall. Place the foam pillow on top of your right shoulder flush with the wall, and place the side of your head snugly against the pillow (Figure 19). Now tilt your head directly sideways to the right, pushing into the foam pillow (Figure 20). Push as hard as you comfortably can, hold for 10

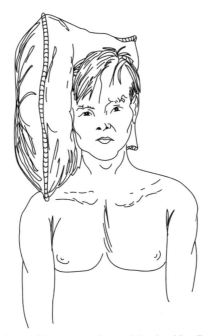

Figure 19 *Place the foam pillow on top of your right shoulder. Push the side of your head firmly against the pillow.*

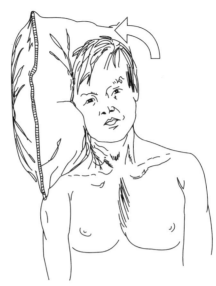

Figure 20   *Push your head into the pillow as hard as you comfortably can. Hold for 10 seconds. Slowly release and relax. Repeat three to five times.*

seconds, then slowly release and relax. Repeat this exercise three to five times per exercise session. Increase as tolerated up to 12 repetitions. Some individuals may only be able to perform this exercise without a pillow; resistance provided by the hand against the side of the face may suffice. Others may only be able to perform the movement against no resistance at all.

Exercise 11: Splenius Capitis and Others on Both Sides

This next exercise is designed to strengthen all of the muscles that tilt the head straight backwards. These lie along the back of the neck on either side of the spine, including the SC. This exercise may be useful for people with anterocollis, as depicted in Chapter 13, Figure 2. Begin by lying on your back on a firm surface with the foam pillow underneath your head (Figure 21). Tilt your head straight backward, pushing into the foam block (Figure 22). Push as hard as you comfortably can, hold for 10 seconds, then slowly release and relax. Repeat this exercise three to five times per exercise session. Increase as tolerated up to 12 repetitions.

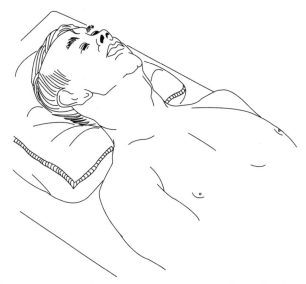

Figure 21 *Lie flat on your back with a foam pillow beneath your head. Tilt your head straight back and push into the foam block.*

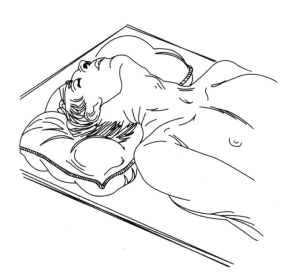

Figure 22 *Push as hard as you can and hold for 10 seconds, and then slowly release and relax. Repeat three to five times.*

Resources

Congratulations! You've just completed the first step in learning to live with dystonia—educating yourself about the disorder. There are other things you can do that are generally helpful. Joining a support group can provide encouragement, camaraderie, and information on the latest medical advances and treatments for dystonia. Having dystonia is not a hopeless situation, and many times others with the disorder enjoy sharing their coping techniques. Maintaining a sense of good general health through diet and exercise will help as well. It's important to maintain contact with your doctor so that an effective treatment strategy can be developed.

ORGANIZATIONS

Listed here are patient organizations that are rich sources of information on dystonias. They offer reading materials, books, and videos on these subjects, and they may assist you in finding a local support group or a specialist who treats dystonia in your area. The names of the organizations are presented in alphabetical order.

The Bachmann-Strauss Dystonia & Parkinson Foundation

From her own suffering as a patient with spasmodic torticollis, Bonnie Strauss was determined to make a difference. Given her family history that her maternal mother and grandmother had Parkinson disease, she had a specific interest in movement disorders, dystonia and Parkinson disease, and the overlap between the two. Her personal dedication led her to create the Annual Dystonia Golf Invitational and 2 years later in 1995 she launched the Bachmann-Strauss Dystonia and Parkinson Foundation (BSDPF).

The BSDPF focuses on finding better treatments and cures for dystonia and Parkinson disease and distributing medical and patient information. The BSDPF is incorporated as an independent non-profit organization headquartered in New York. It works with scientists, clinicians, hospitals, and research centers nationally and internationally. It awards grants for research, creates forums for scientific dialogue, and helps patients and their families better understand dystonia and Parkinson disease.

To date, the BSDPF has raised more than $20 million and funded more than 180 research grants around the world, increasing the understanding of these devastating diseases and producing several new treatments. The foundation has advanced progress in finding better treatments and cures by promoting collaborative efforts among noted scientists and clinicians through the foundation's annual Think Tank. In addition, an annual free symposium provides information to patients, families, and health care providers about the latest treatments and research.

The BSDPF's Scientific Advisory Board (SAB) is led by Dr. Ted Dawson, Director of the Parkinson's Disease and Movement Disorder Center at the Johns Hopkins University School of Medicine. All grant research requests are reviewed by this board, with funding ultimately decided by the BSDPF board of directors based on the recommendations of the SAB.

From its initial program of funding for a yearly grant of $50,000, the foundation has grown and expanded its portfolio of funding to include the following three areas: research grants, identified areas of research focus, and the Center of Excellence. Research funded by BSDPF over the course of the last decade and a half has resulted in finding and perfecting animal models of various forms of dystonia, cloning the DYT-1 gene, and development of its first genetically-altered mouse, a DYT-1 model in the roundworm. These models allowed rapid screening for possible treatment for dystonia drugs. BSDPF has also recognized the challenges of fragmented clinical care by initiating the development of the Dystonia Center of Excellence. Such centers bring together the clinical and research know-how needed to catalyze major advances in scientific understanding and translate them into new treatments. The first Bachmann-Strauss Dystonia Center of Excellence opened at Beth Israel Medical Center in New York City in October 2009.

In addition to funding research, the foundation focuses on educational opportunities for the scientific community and the lay public.

Beginning in 2001, each year the BSDPF has brought together pre-eminent researchers and clinicians from around the world who are experts in the fields of dystonia and Parkinson disease to develop future goals to accelerate the pace of research and to make recommendations of how BSDPF can best continue to impact progress.

The symposiums organized by the foundation for patients, their families, and caregivers provide an important forum for discussions about current and new treatments and therapies. The organization has also published brochures and other materials related to dystonia and Parkinson disease. More information about treatments, research, patient care, and other activities of the BSDPF can be obtained from their Web site (www.dystonia-parkinson.org) or by phone at 212.682.9900.

The Benign Essential Blepharospasm Research Foundation

One of the oldest patient organizations is the Benign Essential Blepharospasm Research Foundation. It was founded in 1981 by Mattie Lou Koster, a dynamic single-minded blepharospasm patient. At the time, there was little awareness of the existence of blepharospasm, leading Mattie Lou to set out to educate the public and create a rallying point for the blepharospasm patients. The organization has grown from a one-woman show to a nationwide well-funded organization with many dedicated volunteers.

The mission of the BEBRF is to fund and promote medical research on the causes and cures of blepharospasm, Meige, and other related disorders of the facial musculature; to provide support, education, and referrals to persons with these disorders; and to disseminate information and serve as an authoritative resource to the medical community and the general public.

Since 1985, the BEBRF has supported and funded medical research into new treatments; pathophysiology; and the genetics involved with focal dystonias, benign essential blepharospasm, Meige, photophobia, dry eye, and apraxia of eyelid opening. The BEBRF Medical Advisory Board is chaired by Dr. Mark Hallett and directs the BEBRF research program.

Blepharospasm/Meige patients volunteer to serve as support group leaders nationally and internationally, helping to provide opportunities for doctors, patients, and their families to share and learn together. Through these times together, patients can discover new treatment options, better ways to cope, and feel that they are not alone.

The BEBRF also strives to provide more information about movement disorders by printing and disseminating educational literature pertaining to BEB/Meige to anyone who seeks such information. The organization also provides a medical CD and DVD library and conducts regional symposiums. Internationally, the BEBRF sponsors international brainstorming workshops for doctors and hosts conferences.

At present, the BEBRF is actively involved in seeking access to better health care on behalf of all dystonia patients through its involvement in the Dystonia Advocacy Network, as well as in the National Institutes of Health's Dystonia Coalition.

Contact the BEBRF at P.O. Box 12468, Beaumont, TX 77726, or call 409–832-0788 or send a fax to 409–832-0890. The official Web site is www.blepharospasm.org and their e-mail is bebrf@blepharospasm.org or bebrf@sbcglobal.net.

The Dystonia Medical Research Foundation

After doctors diagnosed their daughter with dystonia, Samuel and Frances Belzberg decided to create the Dystonia Medical Research Foundation (DMRF) in 1976 in British Columbia. Their main goals were to give assistance to patients with dystonia and their families. Since then, the DMRF has grown considerably and currently has a membership of about 38,000 people. In addition to its original objectives, the organization also aims to support studies on cures for dystonia and to improve general knowledge of the disorder.

As the largest organization, the DMRF provides both support for the patient and funding for research. The DMRF is advised on what research projects to fund by the foundation's Medical and Scientific Director, Mahlon DeLong, MD, of Emory University, the foundation's full time Science Officer, Jan Teller, PhD, MA, and the Medical and Scientific Advisory Council, a group of specialists in subjects such as neurology and genetics. In part, these specialists choose studies based on whether they will generate results that lead to more successful treatments or cures for dystonia.

In 2006 the DMRF founded the Cure Dystonia Initiative (CDI) to further advance research on dystonia treatments in the hope of developing more cures. Notably, the CDI is based on similar programs advocating different diseases or disorders, with an emphasis on the business aspect of researching and producing cures.

Research projects that are being funded by the DMRF in 2009 include "Identification of Novel Drug Targets for DYT1 Dystonia" by Biofocus DPI and "Dopamine Neuron Development in a Novel Zebrafish Model of DYT1 Dystonia" by Edward Burton, PhD, of the University of Pittsburgh.

The DMRF also offers 2-year fellowships to those who wish to begin careers in treating or researching dystonia. Like several other organizations involved with the Dystonia Advocacy Network, the DMRF is also involved in increasing awareness of dystonia on the congressional level. It advocates, among other things, continued federal funding for the National Institutes of Health and for Medicare and Medicaid to provide insurance coverage for procedures relating to dystonia and other movement disorders.

Another goal of the DMRF is to provide support to patients with dystonia. To this effect, their Web site (www.dystonia-foundation. org) features a database of physicians that specialize in treating movement disorders, links to a variety of support groups, advice on how to cope with dystonia both physically and mentally, and information about the disorder aimed specifically at teens and children.

It publishes *Dystonia Dialogue* 3 times a year, reaching about 40,000 people, including doctors, patients, and volunteer groups. In addition to regular patient education symposiums, the DMRF has 50 support groups throughout the country and offers online forums on MySpace, Facebook, Twitter, Ning, and the Online Dystonia Bulletin Board. To learn more about dystonia, contact the Dystonia Medical Research Foundation at One East Wacker Drive, Suite 2810, Chicago, IL 60601–1905, 1–800–377–3978, or online at www.dystonia-foundation.org.

The National Spasmodic Dysphonia Association

Dr. Daniel Truong began his first job in Michigan in 1988. Throughout the course of his study on the use of botulinum toxin for treating spasmodic dysphonia, he realized that the disorder was largely unknown to the medical community. In order to bring about more awareness of spasmodic dysphonia, Dr. Truong proposed the idea of a patient organization to three of his most dynamic patients: Lawrence Kolasa, Rick Johnston, and Paula Mahinske. Together they launched the National Spasmodic Dysphonia Association (NSDA), with the support of Dot Sowerby in North Carolina and Midge Kovacs in New York. Lawrence Kolasa acts as president and was instrumental in getting NSDA to its current stage. At the time, Midge Kovac's newsletter "Our Voice" became the unofficial initial publication for the NSDA. On March 9, 1991, Dr. Daniel Truong organized the first NSDA patients' conference in Irvine, California. Surprisingly, more than 100 patients from nearly 30 states participated. Also at this conference the first full NSDA board meeting was able to meet and the NSDA was born.

The mission of the NSDA is to advance medical research into the causes of and treatments for spasmodic dysphonia, to promote physician and public awareness of the disorder, and to provide support to those affected by spasmodic dysphonia.

The NSDA has produced the award-winning diagnostic video, "What is Spasmodic Dysphonia?" starring honorary board member Chip Hanauer. Chip, a Motorsports Hall of Fame speedboat racer, has elevated awareness of SD to a new level by using every interview as an opportunity to inform the public of his SD. Similarly, Diane Rehm, also an honorary member of the board, has used her National Public Radio talk show and her autobiography, *Finding My Words*, as platforms from which to educate the public about the disorder.

In 1999 the book *Speechless: Living with Spasmodic Dysphonia* was published to celebrate the tenth anniversary of the NSDA. It is the biography of NSDA Board Member Dot Sowerby's experience with SD.

The NSDA promotes the understanding of SD among speech and medical professionals by the writing and/or approval of scientific brochures, materials, and articles for the newsletter and assisting with medical conventions, including selection and material distribution. The NSDA also provides research grants and encourages SD researchers to apply for grant programs.

The NSDA's address is 300 Park Boulevard, Suite 301, Itasca, IL 60413. Their telephone number is 800–795-6732 and their fax is 630–250-4505. You can find them on line at www.dysphonia.org.

The National Spasmodic Torticollis Association

The National Spasmodic Torticollis Association (NSTA) was founded in 1980 by Project S.T. with the goal of making the public aware of spasmodic torticollis and enabling patients with this disorder to share their experiences and overcome the difficulties associated with their condition. Originally located in Michigan, the NSTA moved its headquarters to Fountain Valley, California, in 1997. With the help of its members, medical professionals, and volunteers, the NSTA has become an international organization and has significantly expanded the services it offers.

With regard to supporting research, the NSTA awards seed grants to projects that focus on dystonic movement disorders and that have the possibility of adding to and understanding the treatment of spasmodic torticollis. The end goal is to support these initial studies so that the researchers can generate helpful results and then apply for larger research grants from other public and private sources.

The NSTA's motto is "Remember...You are not alone." Accordingly, the NSTA offers patient services such as a support line (1–800-HURTFUL), a network of support groups and patient contact volunteers, quarterly newsmagazines, and a Web site and message forum (www.torticollis.org). The support line is especially helpful in providing emotional support to callers. Often, patients with dystonia struggle with their symptoms and limitations and may feel isolated because of them. The NSTA's objective is to help these patients by connecting them with other people who understand their experience, so that they can feel less alone.

The NSTA also hosts yearly symposiums in different locations around the United States and invites doctors specializing in movement disorders in the area to speak to the attendees. Another benefit of such symposiums is the inclusion of open topic meetings for people with spasmodic torticollis, as well as for their family, friends, and caretakers. These provide the opportunity for attendees to share their experiences and gain new knowledge and support from other people.

Moreover, Dixie Carter, who starred in the sitcom *Designing Women*, and Jerry West, a former manager of the Los Angeles Lakers, have been featured in two public service announcement videos produced by the NSTA. These PSAs have been aired many times and have proved to be a valuable way of spreading information about spasmodic torticollis.

Additionally, the NSTA is involved with the Dystonia Advocacy Network, along several other organizations. The intent of this group is to unite the differing ideas and missions of all the organizations it in order to make members of Congress aware of dystonia and movement disorders. Ultimately, the DAC aims to develop and implement a legislative and policy agenda to better the lives of people with dystonia.

The NSTA's address is 9920 Talbert Ave, Fountain Valley, CA 92708. Send an e-mail to NSTAmail@aol.com or call 714-378-7837.

ST/Dystonia

The ST/Dystonia group first met in February, 1987 in Milwaukee, Wisconsin, at St. Mary's Hospital on the Lake. Approximately 25 people attended and no one really knew anyone else. Nevertheless, it was a great meeting and they all decided to continue to meet every month. After about a year or so they adopted the name Spasmodic Torticollis of Wisconsin. In 1989 the group was incorporated under that name and eventually became a 501(c)3 nonprofit association in 1991.

As the years went by it became one of the largest support groups operating in the United States, with attendance averaging between 40 and 60 people. In the summer months Spasmodic Torticollis of Wisconsin would host a picnic complete with free hot dogs, hamburgers, bratwurst, beer, and soda and a three-piece band. At one point, 410 people attended one of these picnics, which was unheard of in those days. Some of the meetings in the cooler months attracted notable speakers, which in turn drew well over 100 people.

In 1998, Spasmodic Torticollis of Wisconsin decided that people with spasmodic torticollis needed more and continual help. Consequently, they made the decision to go national and shortened their organization's name to "ST/Dystonia." The organization has since expanded the benefits it offers, including a 24-page quarterly newsmagazine, yearly symposium, toll-free phone number, international Web site, great brochures, disability kit, tweener letter (in-between the newsmagazines), and discussion forums on the Web. In the near future ST/Dystonia also plans to release a 20-minute DVD containing physical therapy exercises.

The main goal of ST/Dystonia is to provide hope for the future for all ST-ers. Its mission statement is "helping people find a faster diagnosis and more effective treatments, thus empowering them to achieve a higher quality of life."

Contact ST/Dystonia at P.O. Box 28, Mukwonago, WI 53149 or info@spasmodictorticollis.org. The official ST/Dystonia Web site is www.spasmodictorticollis.org and their toll-free number is 1–888-445-4588.

We Move (Worldwide Education and Awareness for Movement Disorders) 204 West 84th Street, New York, NY 10024; Phone: 800–437-MOV2; Fax: 212–875-8389; e-mail: wemove@wemove.org; Web site: www.wemove.org

OTHER RESOURCES

Books

Jean-Pierre Bleton. *Spasmodic Torticollis Handbook of Rehabilitative Physiotherapy.* (Paris, France: Editions Frison-Roche, 1994.)

Video

National Spasmodic Torticollis Association. *Physical Therapy and Exercises for Spasmodic Torticollis.* http://www.torticollis.org/PTvideo.html.

Glossary

Abductor: Muscles that move two body parts away from each other.

Acetylcholine: A *neurotransmitter* used extensively within the central nervous system and the parasympathetic nervous system.

Adductors: Muscles that move two body parts closer together.

Advil: A brand name over-the-counter pain medication; generic name *ibuprofen.*

Agonist: For the purposes of this book, this is the primary muscle or set of muscles that is involuntarily contracting and pulling the head and neck into abnormal posture in *spasmodic torticollis.*

Aleve: A brand name over-the-counter pain medication; generic name *naproxen.*

Alpha-receptor agonist: A pharmaceutical category of medications that may be used to treat muscle spasms and pain.

Alprazolam: The generic name for *Xanax.*

Amitriptyline: The generic name for *Elavil.*

Anoxia: Any state of oxygen deprivation; may lead to brain damage.

Antagonist: For the purposes of this book, this is any muscle or set of muscles that can oppose the pulling force of *agonists* to move the head and neck back toward normal position.

Anterocollis: Forward tilting of the head, tucking the chin into the chest. This is the most difficult abnormal head posture to treat medically.

Anticholinergic: A pharmaceutical category of medications that may be used to treat movement disorders. These medications inhibit the actions of *acetylcholine* in some locations and thus diminish the effects of the *parasympathetic nervous system.*

Antidepressant: A medication used to treat depression and also pain.

Antipsychotic: Synonymous with *neuroleptic*. A psychiatric medication used to treat disorders characterized by hallucinations, delusions, or agitated behavior. Most antipsychotics block the action of the brain chemical *dopamine*. They may cause movement disorders.

Artane: An *anticholinergic* medication that may be used to treat movement disorders; generic name *trihexphenidyl*.

Ativan: A sedative medication of the *benzodiazepine* class that may be used to treat *movement disorders*; generic name *lorazepam*.

Atlanto-axial dislocation: A slippage of the two topmost cervical vertebrae that results in abnormal head posture.

Atrophy: Muscle shrinkage and deterioration. This will occur if the motor nerve that delivers signals to a muscle is cut, chronically compressed, or otherwise disrupted.

Axon: The long wirelike process extending outward from a neuron through which the neuron sends out its electrical and chemical signals.

Baclofen: An antispasicidy medication that enhances the activity of *GABA*.

Ballism: Large, dramatic involuntary movements such as swinging the arm up and down. Can be considered a type of dyskinesia.

Basal ganglia: Several berry-sized clusters of neurons deep within the brain. They are an integral part of the extrapyramidal motor system. They receive and integrate the varied sensory input information and use it to modulate the output of the pyramidal motor system.

Basal ganglia disorders: This term encompasses most *movement disorders*. Most such disorders have their primary site of abnormality in the *basal ganglia*.

Benadryl: A medication with *anticholinergic* properties that can be used to treat acute *dystonia* or *dyskinesia*; generic name *diphenhydramine*.

Benzodiazepine: A pharmaceutical category of sedative medications that may be used to treat movement disorders.

Benztropine mesylate: The generic name for *Cogentin*.

Blepharospasm: A focal dystonia affecting the facial muscles that squeeze the eyelids closed.

Botox: A brand name of *botulinum toxin* type A.

Botulinum toxin: The nerve toxin produced by the bacterium *Clostridium botulinum*. It is the most commonly used *chemodenervation* medication.

Botulism: A muscle paralyzing disease caused by infection with the bacterium *Clostridium botulinum* through a wound or by ingestion of its toxin in spoiled food.

Bupropion: The generic name of *Wellbutrin*.

Carbidopa: One of the ingredients of *Sinemet*. It protects the active ingredient, *levodopa*, from becoming metabolized before it can enter the brain.

Catapress: A medication in the *alpha-receptor agonist* class that may be used to treat muscle spasms and pain; generic name *clonidine*.

Central nervous system: For purposes of this book, this includes the brain and spinal cord.

Cervical dystonia: Synonymous with spasmodic torticollis; a *neurological* disorder that results in an involuntary turning or twisting of the head and neck, forcing them to assume an abnormal posture.

Cervicalgia: Neck pain.

Cervical spine: The portion of the spinal column in the neck.

Cervix: The neck.

Chemodenervation: The injections of a medication into a muscle or nerve to either destroy the nerve or disrupt its connections to the muscle. The targeted muscle then becomes weakened or paralyzed.

Chorea: Dance-like involuntary movements, can be considered a type of dyskinesia.

Clonazepam: The generic name for *Klonopin*.

Clonidine: The generic name for *Catapress*.

Clostridium botulinum: The species of bacteria that produces *botulinum toxin*.

CNS: See central nervous system.

Cogentin: An *anticholinergic* medication used to treat *movement disorders*. The generic name is *benztropine mesylate*.

Compazine: A medication that blocks the action of *dopamine*. It can cause transient acute *dystonia* or *dyskinesia*. Rarely, it can lead to a permanent movement disorder. The generic name is *prochlorperazine*.

Computed tomography: A computer-assisted X-ray imaging technique.

CT: Computed tomography.

Cymbalta: A *selective norepinephrine and serotonin reuptake inhibitor.* This medication can be used as an antidepressant or a pain reliever.

Dantrium: The generic name for *Dantrolene.*

Dantrolene: An antispasticity medication that works inside muscle tissue. The generic name is *dantrium.*

Deep brain stimulation: The surgical implantation of a battery-driven device that disrupts the electrical signals of the *basal ganglia* and *extrapyramidal motor system* by means of electrode wires that are inserted into the brain. It is used mainly to treat the symptoms of severe *Parkinson disease,* generalized dystonia, and a few other dystonias.

Diazepam: The generic name for *Valium.*

Diphenhydramine: The generic name for *Benadryl.*

Dopamine: One of the principal *neurotransmitters* of the *basal ganglia* and *extrapyramidal motor system.* Drugs or medical conditions that disrupt the activity of dopamine may cause movement disorders. Some drugs that modify dopamine activity may be used to treat movement disorders.

Dopamine-responsive dystonia: A small percentage of movement disorders (other than *Parkinson disease*) that improve with the administration of *Sinemet* or *dopamine agonists.*

Duloxetine: The generic name for *Cymbalta.*

Dyskinesia: Involuntary movement of one or more body parts. It often coexists with dystonia in the same body part. It is a frequent manifestation of movement disorders. Can be composed of dystonia, chorea or ballistic movements.

Dysport: A brand name of *botulinum toxin* type A, marketed in Europe and in the United States.

Dystonia: Sustained involuntary increased muscle tone in one or more body parts. This often results in abnormal posture of the affected part. It is a frequent manifestation of movement disorders.

Effexor: A *selective norepinephrine and serotonin reuptake inhibitor.* This medication can be used for pain control or depression.

Elavil: A *tricyclic antidepressant* that has some *anticholinergic* properties. It can be used to treat the pain associated with neurologic disorders and may mildly diminish *dystonia.* The generic name is *amitriptyline.*

Electromyography (EMG): A diagnostic technique used to monitor and record the electrical activity in contracting muscles. It can also be used to guide the placement of *chemodenervation* injections.

Encephalitis: Any infection or inflammation affecting the brain.

Extrapyramidal disorders: This term encompasses most *movement disorders*. The primary site of abnormality is usually in the *basal ganglia*.

Extrapyramidal motor system: A subsystem of the motor system in the CNS. The extrapyramidal system controls and modulates the output of the pyramidal system, acting as a "fine tuner" of movements and preventing excessive movements. The basal ganglia are an integral part of the extrapyramidal system.

Foramina: "Windows." These are gaps between each of the *vertebrae* through which nerve roots containing motor and sensory components pass. The foramina are common sites at which such nerves may become compressed or "pinched."

GABA: Gamma-amino butyric acid. A *neurotransmitter* in the brain and spinal cord that has mainly inhibitory properties.

Geste antagoniste: "Sensory trick." This usually consists of brushing one's fingers or hand against the face and neck, and it may help to bring the head position in spasmodic torticollis back to normal.

Haldol: An antipsychotic or *neuroleptic* medication that can cause dystonia. The generic name is haloperidol.

Haloperidol: The generic neame for *Haldol.*

Honeymoon period: A brief period of time, usually after awakening, during which symptoms of spasmodic torticollis are diminished.

Hydrocodone: A narcotic drug that is an ingredient in *Vicodin* and other pain medications.

Ibuprofen: The generic name for *Advil, Motrin,* and other brand name pain medications.

Idiopathic: A descriptive term for any medical condition that seems to arise of its own accord, with no discernible inciting cause.

Imipramine: The generic name for *Tofranil.*

Involuntary movement: A movement performed automatically without knowledge or ability.

Klonopin: A sedative medication in the *benzodiazepine* class that may be used to treat *movement disorders*. The generic name is *clonazepam*.

Laterocollis: Sideways tilting of the head, moving one ear closer to the shoulder on the same side.

Levator scapuli: Neck muscle whose main action is to lift the shoulder blade upward and elevate the shoulder.

Levodopa: An active ingredient in *Sinemet* and other medications for *Parkinson disease*. It supplies *dopamine* to the brain.

Lidocaine: An anesthetic agent that can be injected into tissues for local pain relief.

Lorazepam: The generic name for *Ativan*.

Magnetic resonance imaging: A computerized medical imaging technique using a magnetic field and radio waves. Abbreviated *MRI*.

Meige syndrome: A focal *dyskinesia* affecting muscles of the face.

Metoclopramide: The generic name for *Reglan*.

Mirapex: A *dopamine agonist*, a medication that mimics the action of *dopamine*. It is usually used to treat Parkinson disease. The generic name is *pramipexole*.

Motor nerves: Nerves that branch off from the spinal cord, emerge from the spinal column through *foramina* between each of the *vertebrae*, and carry signals for contraction and movement out to the muscles.

Motor system: Those parts of the brain and spinal cord concerned with moving the muscles and controlling those movements. This can also include motor nerves carrying signals to the muscles.

Motrin: A brand name over-the-counter pain medication.

Movement disorder: Any neurologic disorder characterized by abnormal posture or movement in one or more body parts.

MRI: Magnetic resonance imaging.

Myobloc: A brand name for *botulinum toxin* type B.

Myotomy: A surgical technique in which specific muscles are cut or removed in order to relieve *dystonia*.

Naproxen sodium: The generic name for *Aleve* and other brand name pain medications.

Nerve root: Nerve structures that are attached to the spinal cord and pass through the *foramina* between each of the *vertebrae*. They contain sensory components bringing input information to the *CNS*, and motor components sending signals for movement out to the muscles.

Neuroleptic: Synonymous with antipsychotic. A psychiatric medication used to treat disorders characterized by hallucinations, delusions, or agitated behavior. Most neuroleptics block the action of the brain chemical dopamine. They may cause movement disorders.

Neuron: A nerve cell that sends and receives signals. These cells are located in the gray matter of the brain, in the basal ganglia, and in the spinal cord.

Neuronox: A brand name of *botulinum toxin* type A available outside the United States.

Neurotransmitter: A chemical that carries a signal from the terminal end of an axon across a small gap to another *neuron* or muscle cell.

Nortriptyline: The generic name for *Pamelor.*

Occupational dystonia: A focal *dystonia* affecting any body part that manifests when performing a particular task.

Ocular dystonia: A focal *dystonia* affecting muscles that move the eyeballs.

Olanzapine: The generic name of *Zyprexa.*

Orbicularis oculi: The facial muscle that squeezes the eyelids closed.

Oromandibular dystonia: A focal *dystonia* affecting muscles of the mouth and jaws.

Pamelor: A *tricyclic antidepressant.* It may be used to treat neurologic causes of pain. The generic name is *nortriptyline.*

Paraplegia: Weakness or paralysis of the two lower limbs due to an injury or other disruption of the spinal cord.

Parasympathetic nervous system: A system of *neurons* and nerves that controls many automatic functions of the body. It uses *acetylcholine* as a *neurotransmitter.*

Paresis: Weakness of one or more body parts due to an injury or disruption of any part of the *motor system.*

Parkinson disease: A movement disorder characterized by tremor of the hands or feet when at rest, increased *resting tone* of muscles resulting in rigidity of the trunk and limbs, a stooped posture, and impairment of balance and gait.

Parlodel: A *dopamine* agonist, a medication that mimics the action of *dopamine*. It is usually used to treat Parkinson disease. The generic name is *bromocriptine*.

Paroxetine: The generic name for *Paxil*.

Paroxysmal Kinesogenic Dyskinesia: an inherited disorder causing episodic dyskinesias to occur at the onset of movement.

Paroxysmal Nonkinesogenic Dyskinesia: an inherited disorder causing episodic dyskinesia not related to movement.

Paroxysmal Exercise Induced Dyskinesia: a disorder causing dyskinesia to occur following a period of exercise.

Paxil: An antidepressant medication in the *SSRI* class. It may help to relieve pain associated with neurologic conditions. The generic name is *paroxetine*.

Peripheral nervous system: This includes motor nerves coming out of the spinal cord, the muscles, and sensory nerves carrying information back to the CNS.

Phenol: A solvent that may be used as a *chemodenervation* agent.

Pramipexole: The generic name for *Mirapex*.

Prochlorperazine: The generic name for *Compazine*.

Prosigne: A brand name of *botulinum toxin* type A available outside the United States.

Pyramidal motor system: A subsystem of the motor system in the CNS. The pyramidal system generates and sends out the primary signal for a group of muscles to contract and cause movement.

Radicular: Anything having to do with the motor and sensory *nerve roots* that pass through the *foramina*. Radicular pain is often felt to radiate along the territory of the sensory component of a *nerve root*. Radicular weakness and *atrophy* can occur among muscles supplied by the motor component of a *nerve root*.

Radiculopathy: Any medical condition that affects a nerve root. Radicular pain is often felt to radiate along the territory of the sensory component of a *nerve root*. Radicular weakness and *atrophy* can occur among muscles supplied by the motor component of a *nerve root*.

Rebound effect: A transient worsening of a medical condition or symptom that may occur if a medication being taken to treat it is abruptly discontinued.

Reglan: A medicine that blocks the action of *dopamine*. It can cause transient acute *dystonia* or *dyskinesia*. Rarely, it can lead to a permanent *movement disorder*. The generic name is *metoclopramide*.

Requip: A *dopamine* agonist, a medication that mimics the action of *dopamine*. It is usually used to treat Parkinson disease. The generic name is *ropinirole*.

Resting tone: The low level of electrical excitation and contraction in which all muscles are maintained during wakefulness. Movement disorders are characterized by abnormalities of resting tone.

Retrocollis: Backward tilting of the head, moving the chin upward, away from the chest.

Rheumatic heart disease: An inflammation of heart tissue associated with a certain bacterial infection. *Sydenham chorea* is one of the long-term sequelae of this condition.

Risperdal: A newer-generation neuroleptic antipsychotic medication that can cause dystonia.

Risperidone: The generic name of *Risperidal*.

Rhizotomy: A surgical technique in which spinal nerve roots are cut in order to relieve pain or muscular *dystonia*.

Ropinirole: The generic name for *Requip*.

Scalenes: Neck muscles whose main action is to pull the neck to the side and tilt the head toward the same side.

Selective peripheral denervation: A surgical technique in which the *motor nerve* branches to specific muscles are cut in order to relieve *dystonia*.

SSRI: See *selective serotonin reuptake inhibitor*.

Selective norepinephrine and serotonin reuptake inhibitors: A subclass of *antidepressant* medications that can be used in pain management.

Selective serotonin reuptake inhibitors: A subclass of *antidepressant* medications that can be used in pain management.

Semispinalis capitis: Neck muscle whose main action is to bend the head and neck backward.

Sensory nerves: Nerves that carry sensory input information from the skin, joints, and muscles to the CNS. They enter the spinal column through the *foramina* between each of the *vertebrae*, merge with the spinal cord, then relay their signals to sensory pathways that reach the brain.

Sensory trick: Same as *geste antagoniste*.

Sertraline: The generic name for *Zoloft*.

Sinemet: A medication that includes the chemicals *carbidopa* and *levodopa*. Its active ingredient is levodopa, which enters the brain and is turned into *dopamine*. It is most often used to treat *Parkinson disease*.

SLE: See *Systemic lupus erythmatosus*.

Spasmodic dysphonia: A focal *dystonia* affecting the vocal cords that impairs the voice.

Spasmodic torticollis: A neurologic movement disorder characterized by abnormal position or tremor of the head and neck. Also known as *cervical dystonia*.

Splenius capitis: Neck muscle whose main action is to bend the head backward and rotate it slightly to the same side.

Splenius cervicis: Neck muscle whose main action is to bend the neck backward.

Sternocleidomastoid: A neck muscle whose main action is to rotate the head toward the opposite side.

Strabismus: A medical condition in which the eyes are misaligned with each other.

Striatum: Certain parts of the basal ganglia that together receive signals via the neurotransmitter *dopamine*; they are important in the control of movement.

Stroke: A neurologic condition caused by a blockage of a brain artery or by bleeding into the brain. The manifestations of a stroke depend on its size and its location in the brain. Occasionally, it can result in a *movement disorder*.

Sydenham chorea: A movement disorder characterized by writhing movements of the limbs. It is a long-term sequela of *rheumatic heart disease*.

Systemic lupus erythematosus: A medical disorder of the body's immune system. The manifestations of this disease are multifold; it can produce *movement disorders* if it affects the brain.

Tardive dyskinesia: A late-onset *movement disorder* that arises months or years after the chronic use of medications that interfere with the action of the brain chemical *dopamine*. It is characterized by increased muscle tone and abnormal movements (such as tremor or writhing) in the affected body parts.

Tardive dystonia: A late-onset *movement disorder* that arises months or years after chronic use of medications that interfere with the action of the brain chemical *dopamine*. It is characterized by increased muscle tone and abnormal posture in the affected body parts, and is usually permanent.

Tension cervicalgia: A temporary disorder characterized by muscle spasms in the neck, aching pain, and a feeling of stiffness. People often hold their head in an abnormal position to avoid pain. This is not a movement disorder.

Thalamotomy: A surgical technique in which a small part of the *basal ganglia* is destroyed. It is used to relieve symptoms of severe *Parkinson disease*.

Thorazine: An older neuroleptic antipsychotic medication that can cause dystonia.

Thioridizine: The generic name of *Thorazine*.

Tizanidine: The generic name for *Zanaflex*.

Tofranil: A *tricyclic antidepressant*. It may be used to treat neurological pain. The generic name is *imipramine*.

Torticollis: "Twisted neck." Often used interchangeably with the term cervical dystonia. An involuntary abnormal posture of the head and neck from any medical condition. This can include developmental or orthopaedic conditions. This term is also used to indicate right or left rotation of the head on its axis.

Trapezius: A neck muscle whose main action is to lift the shoulder upwards.

Trauma: Physical injury to any body part from an external source.

Tricyclic antidepressant: A subclass of *antidepressants* that can be used for pain management.

Trihexphenidyl: The generic name for *Artane*.

Valium: A sedative medication in the *benzodiazepine* class that may be used to treat *movement disorders*.

Venlafaxine: The generic name of *Effexor*.

Vertebra: One of the bones stacked upon one another that form the spinal column.

Vertebrae: Plural of vertebra.

Vicodin: A brand name pain medication containing a combination of the narcotic hydrocodone and acetominophen.

Wellbutrin: A *selective norepinephrine and serotonin reuptake inhibitor (SNRI)*. This medication can be used as an antidepressant or pain medication.

Whiplash: A term used to describe the type of neck injury that occurs with a sudden acceleration and deceleration of the body, causing the head and neck to flex back and forth rapidly. This may occur in a motor vehicle collision.

Wilson disease: A metabolic disorder in which the normal metabolism of the trace mineral copper is disrupted. One of its manifestations is as a movement disorder.

Writer's cramp: A focal *dystonia* affecting arm and hand muscles that manifests during writing or similar tasks.

Wry-neck: In this book, this term is synonymous with *tension cervicalgia*.

Xanax: A sedative medication in the benzodiazepine class that may be used to treat *movement disorders*.

Xeomin: A brand name of *botulinum toxin* type A available outside the United States.

Zanaflex: A medication in the *alpha-receptor agonist* class that may be used to treat muscle spasms and pain. The generic name is *tizanidine*.

Zoloft: An *antidepressant* medication in the *SSRI* class. It may help relieve pain associated with neurological conditions. The generic name is *sertraline*.

Zyprexa: A newer generation neuroleptic antipsychotic medication that can cause dystonia.

About the Authors

Daniel Truong underwent his medical training at the Ludwig Albert University in Freiburg, Germany. He completed residency training in both Neurology and Psychiatry in Germany before moving to the United States, where he completed a neurology residency at the Medical University of South Carolina. He received three years of fellowship training in Parkinson Disease and other movement disorders at Columbia University, New York, and the National Hospital for Nervous Disease at Queen Square in London, where he studied under the two founders of the field, Professor Stanley Fahn and the late Prof. David Marsden. Dr. Truong also founded the Parkinson's and Movement Disorders Program at the University of California, Irvine and, together with his patients, founded the National Spasmodic Dysphonia Association—now in its twentieth year—where he continues as an honorary board member.

Over the past 25 years, Dr. Truong has participated in numerous multicenter clinical trials examining novel medications for the treatment of movement disorders, and was one of the early investigators of botulinum toxin prior to its approval by the U.S. Food and Drug Administration. He is known for the development of an animal model for myoclonus, a movement disorder that may occur following a period of hypoxia. He developed the Truong and Fahn Myoclonus Rating Scale to measure the disorder in humans. Dr. Truong serves on the editorial board of many medical journals and has published more than 120 papers and 6 books. He has spoken worldwide on different topics related to Parkinson disease and other movement disorders and served as the editor of the textbook *International Neurology*. Dr. Truong serves on different capacities in many international neurological organizations.

Dr. Truong currently practices medicine in Orange County, California. He currently resides in Huntington Beach, California, with his wife and three children.

Mayank Pathak, a graduate of the George Washington University School of Medicine, completed residency training at the University of California, Irvine, followed by two fellowships, one in spinal cord medicine at the Veteran's Administration Hospital in Long Beach, California, and another in neurological rehabilitation at the University of California, Los Angeles. He joined the Parkinson's and Movement Disorders Institute in Orange County, California in 1998, involving himself in both the treatment and research of dystonia. He co-authored *The Spasmodic Torticollis Handbook*, has published a number of papers and book chapters in this field, and creates medical anatomical illustrations for his own publications. Dr. Pathak lives in Orange County with his wife and two children.

Karen Frei is a graduate of Jefferson Medical College. She completed neurology training at the Barrow's Neurological Institute in Phoenix, Arizona. She then traveled to Bethesda, Maryland, and finished a clinical research fellowship at the National Institutes of Health. She has been practicing neurology with a subspecialty of movement disorders at the Parkinson's and Movement Disorders Institute over the past 10 years. She enjoys serving as the medical editor for the National Spasmodic Torticollis Association and is dedicated to helping her patients. She is the author of several books, chapters, and articles and is an acclaimed speaker. She resides in Alta Loma, California, with her family, two shih tzu puppies, Lucy and Lizzy, and a Siamese cat named Fortune Cookie.

Index

Note: Page numbers followed by 'f' and 't' indicate figures and tables, respectively.